COMMUNICABLE
AND NON-COMMUNICABLE
DISEASE BASICS

COMMUNICABLE
AND NON-COMMUNICABLE
DISEASE
BASICS

A PRIMER

Madeline M. Hurster

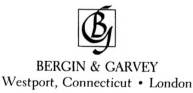

BERGIN & GARVEY
Westport, Connecticut • London

Library of Congress Cataloging-in-Publication Data

Hurster, Madeline M., 1925–
    Communicable and non-communicable disease basics : a primer /
Madeline M. Hurster.
        p. cm.
    Includes bibliographical references.
    ISBN 0–89789–507–X (alk. paper). — ISBN 0–89789–508–8 (pbk. :
alk. paper)
        1. Diseases—Causes and theories of causation. 2. Communicable
diseases. 3. Constitutional diseases. I. Title.
    RB151.H87 1997
    616—dc21   97–12667

British Library Cataloguing in Publication Data is available.

Library of Congress Catalog Card Number: 97–12667
ISBN: 0–89789–507–X
        0–89789–508–8 (pbk.)

First published in 1997

Bergin & Garvey, 88 Post Road West, Westport, CT 06881
An imprint of Greenwood Publishing Group, Inc.

Printed in the United States of America

The paper used in this book complies with the
Permanent Paper Standard issued by the National
Information Standards Organization (Z39.48–1984).

10 9 8 7 6 5 4 3 2 1

Every reasonable effort has been made to trace the owners of copyright materials in this book, but in some instances this has proven impossible. The
author and publisher will be glad to receive information leading to more
complete acknowledgments in subsequent printings of the book and in the
meantime extend their apologies for any omissions.

CONTENTS

ILLUSTRATIONS

CHARTS

FIGURES

PREFACE

This text is designed to provide a framework for understanding the disease process in humans. By means of this framework, the reader will become aware of the basic differences between communicable and non-communicable diseases with respect to their genesis and the body's response to them, as well as how the individual, community, and government can assist in the prevention, control, and management of each group of diseases. The text is primarily intended for undergraduate students in allied health professional preparation programs, and for undergraduates in early childhood/elementary education preparation programs. It will also be of value to students in a personal health course.

Since students in the aforementioned disciplines will not be engaged in the "laying-on of hands," nor be responsible for diagnosing and prescribing for illnesses, their need to know specific causes, symptoms, and treatments is not of prime importance. As interesting and worthwhile as such information may be, it is soon forgotten unless the student has reason to apply it. By providing a conceptual framework to comprehend disease, this text will allow the student to make appropriate connections between the disease process and his or her own life, as well as the lives of his or her clients or students. Since disease is a universal phenomenon, this text will serve a useful purpose wherever the aforementioned programs are offered.

1

FRAMEWORK FOR UNDERSTANDING THE DISEASE PROCESS

DISEASE DEFINED

Disease has been viewed as the opposite of wellness or health. Implicit in this contrast is the assumption that when someone is well, he or she is free from disease; yet many who are apparently "well" may be harboring the seeds of disease. So then, what exactly is a disease?

From a physiological/medical point of view, disease refers specifically to the malfunctioning of a body part. The focus, in this case, is on a body part. From a sociological standpoint, disease refers to the malfunctioning of a community, and how it impacts the health of its members. Anthropologists may view disease as a culturally determined phenomenon that affects health. From yet another point of view, disease may be regarded as something that causes a person to function at less than his or her optimum capacity. This is, of course, a purely subjective evaluation. Few of us truly know what our optimum is. History is replete with examples of people who have managed to accomplish prodigious tasks in spite of severe limitations. Beethoven, who was totally deaf for the last ten years of his life, is a prime example of such a person.

So we are saying that disease cannot be defined one-dimensionally; it has many ramifications. Whether discussing communicable or non-communicable diseases, we need to keep this in mind. Disease not only involves the interaction of body part with disease agent, but also the interactions of body part with body part, and the body with the several environments in which we live. The ability to adapt to these interactions becomes the measure of one's state of health, or state of disease.

To clarify how these interactions work, a set of laws, or canons, has been formulated. Known as the Biological Laws of Disease, they serve to explain the relationships between disease agent, host (or target of the disease agent), and environment, and also to incorporate the concept that disease is a multidimensional phenomenon.

BIOLOGICAL LAWS OF DISEASE

Whether considering a communicable or non-communicable disease, the following laws, or canons, may be applied:

1. Disease results when there is an imbalance between the host and the agent.
2. The nature and extent of the imbalance are determined by the nature and characteristics of the host and agent.
3. These characteristics are largely governed by conditions of the environment.

Biological Law 1: Disease Results When There Is an Imbalance Between the Host and the Agent

This law implies that there is an interaction between two entities: the *host* and the *agent,* and that when the agent is the stronger or more dominant force, a disease state will result. The host may be defined as the recipient of the disease, or as the person who succumbs to the agent and develops a disease. In the case of a communicable disease, the agent is always the cause. In non-communicable disease, the term agent refers to the factor or factors contributing or predisposing to the onset or development of the disease.

For our purposes, the host is always *man.* The agent, on the other hand, is either a *pathogen,* or *germ,* in the case of a communicable disease; or a *genetic, behavioral,* or *environmental factor* in the case of a non-communicable disease.

Biological Law 2: The Nature and Extent of the Imbalance Are Determined by the Nature and Characteristics of the Host and Agent

Nature of the imbalance refers to the *kind* of disease that has resulted from the interaction between host and agent. That is, has the imbalance led to a communicable disease or a non-communicable disease; and specifically, to *which* disease?

The term *extent* refers to the *severity* of the imbalance, or how serious a case of the disease has the host come down with?

Nature and characteristics of the host refers to the host's level of resistance in the case of a communicable disease, or to the number of contributing or predisposing factors to which the host is exposed in the case of a non-communicable disease. That is, if the host is subject to several contributing factors, he or she is considered to be at greater risk of developing a non-communicable disease.

When considering a communicable disease, the term *nature and characteristics of the agent* refers to the ability of the agent to enter and lodge in the body, multiply, and spread throughout the body, thus creating a disease state in the host. Entering, lodging, multiplying, and spreading are characteristics that may be subsumed under the heading of *infectivity*. Creating a disease state may also be referred to as *pathogenicity*. Infectivity and pathogenicity are generic characteristics of pathogens.

When considering a non-communicable disease, the term *nature and characteristics of the agent*, refers to how modifiable, pervasive, and prevalent it is.

Biological Law 3: These Characteristics Are Largely Governed by Conditions of the Environment

Environment refers to such factors as temperature, moisture, exposure to sunlight, and availability of oxygen, as well as crowding, level of sanitation, noise, and poverty. These factors impact the ability of both the host and agent to survive. With regard to the host, they may either increase or diminish the ability to ward off invasion by a pathogen. In the case of the agent, they may either enhance or reduce its ability to induce a disease state in the host.

The essence of these three laws is that in any disease state, there are always three players: (1) the person or host who is the target of disease, and who may or may not succumb to it; (2) the agent, which is either the direct cause of disease or a contributing or predisposing factor to its onset; and (3) the environment, which may either enhance or reduce the host's chances of resisting disease, or the agent's ability to induce a disease state.

BODY'S LINES OF DEFENSE

Any quick observation of those around us will indicate that most people are reasonably well, most of the time. Being reasonably well means that for the most part we are able to perform our daily tasks with a fair amount of efficiency. And we are able to do this in spite of the fact that we are constantly being exposed to disease agents of one sort or another. Clearly, some phenomenon must be at work to prevent our falling ill much more frequently than we do. The ability to resist disease agents is a function of the body's three lines of defense. The first two are usually present in all people from birth on, and could be considered universal features of man. They function automatically, so we do not have to consciously call them into play to ward off a disease agent. Another characteristic is that they will respond to any agent; their action could be described as indiscriminate. In contrast, the third line of defense is not considered universal so far as its presence in man is concerned, and its action is not indiscriminate.

The Body's First Line of Defense

The body's first line of defense serves as the outermost barrier to a disease agent. It consists of a number of structures and reflexes, whose primary role is to prevent the disease agent from entering and getting a foothold in the body. Foremost among these is the *skin*. When the skin remains intact (unbroken) and clean, it serves as an excellent barrier to disease agents. The tiny hairs, or *cilia*, which line the nasal and respiratory passages, filter out disease particles from the air that we inhale. *Mucous membranes* also line these passages, providing a sticky surface to which foreign particles (including disease agents) may adhere, thus preventing their further penetration of the body. *Reflexes*, such as tearing and blinking of the eyes, sneezing, coughing, and vomiting, also either prevent entry of foreign particles or expel them as quickly as possible. These first-line defenses are usually present in everyone, function automatically on our behalf, and respond to any foreign agent that attempts to enter the body.

The Body's Second Line of Defense

Once a disease agent has succeeded in getting past the first-line defenses, the second-line defenses come into play. These, like the first line, are usually present in all people, act automatically when the need arises, and respond to any foreign agent that enters the body. Two major systems of the body are involved as second-line defenses: the *reticulo-endothelial system* and the *lymphatic system*.

The reticulo-endothelial system is made up of cells that have the ability to destroy by ingestion, or phagocytosis, such disease agents as bacteria and viruses. These cells are of two types: (1) phagocytic cells of the bone marrow, spleen, liver, and lymph nodes, called *histiocytes*; and (2) the white blood cells, or *leukocytes*, of the circulatory system, also referred to as *monocytes*. When histiocytes and monocytes encounter a foreign agent, they are activated and become *macrophages*. As macrophages, they are larger and more phagocytic than they were before encountering the foreign agent. Another component of the reticulo-endothelial system is *interferon*, a protein which is produced in response to and designed to combat viruses.

The lymphatic system is an accessory system which filters foreign agents out of tissue and the blood. Thus, it works in conjunction with the reticulo-endothelial system in combatting those agents that have succeeded in getting past the first-line defenses. The lymphatic system is made up of lymph, lymph ducts, and lymph nodes.

Lymph is a watery substance, very much like blood plasma. Lymph ducts are the conduits through which lymph flows, and lymph nodes are collecting places for foreign agents absorbed by the lymph from tissue and blood. The major lymph nodes are located in the neck, the groin, and under the armpits. Swollen lymph nodes may be a sign of infection.

In summary, second-line defenses come into play when the pathogen, or foreign agent, has succeeded in entering the body and is attempting to find a lodging place where it may multiply, and from which it may spread. The second-line defenses respond by focusing on the invasion site; surrounding the invader, thus inhibiting its ability to spread and find nutrition; and finally by phagocytizing the invader. The reticulo-endothelial and lymphatic systems work in concert, with their overall goal being to halt the progress of the foreign agent. They respond to any foreign agent; that is, their response may be described as non-specific. In addition, their response is automatic.

The Body's Third Line of Defense

This line of defense consists of *antibodies*, protein substances or globulins which derive from two kinds of cells: B lymphocytes and T lymphocytes. These cells are formed in bone marrow and come into play when a foreign agent, or pathogen, not only succeeds in evading the first-line defenses, but also begins to gain a foothold in the body; that is, to lodge, multiply, and spread. Both varieties of lymphocytes are found in the blood. When B cells and T cells interact with a pathogen or foreign agent, they produce antibodies. Unlike the previously described lines of defense, which are usually present in all people and non-specific in their response to foreign agents, antibodies must be acquired and are specific in their response. This means that an antibody will only take action against the antigen that initially stimulated the antibody's production. Thus, antibodies produced against one disease will not protect the host from another disease.

How Antibodies Work

There are two general kinds of antigen/antibody reactions. One results directly in destruction of the antigen; the other causes the antigen to become more susceptible to phagocytosis by the cells of the reticulo-endothelial and lymphatic systems. *Lysis* is the process in which the pathogen's cell walls are dissolved by actions of antibodies and complement, a substance found in the plasma. When this occurs, the pathogen is no longer viable as a disease-producing agent.

There are four different antigen/antibody reactions which are designed to render the antigen more susceptible to phagocytosis: neutralization, agglutination, precipitation, and opsonization. *Neutralization* occurs in response to both toxins and viruses. The toxin and/or virus is covered by the antibody and thereby rendered incapable of acting on the body. *Agglutination* results in the clumping of the antigenic cells, thus making it impossible for them to enter tissue and create a disease state. *Precipitation* decreases the antigen's ability to remain soluble, thereby lessening its ability to circulate throughout the body, and *opsonization* is the process in which the antigen becomes coated with antibody. Each of these reactions facilitates destruction of the antigen by the cells of the reticulo-endothelial and lymphatic systems.

Autoimmune Response

A basic function of antibodies is to distinguish between foreign matter or pathogens and the normal cells of the body. A complex series of responses enables the antibody to do this. Occasionally, however, this ability to differentiate between the antigen and the normal cell (which the antibody should be protecting) goes awry, and the antibody proceeds to attack normal cell tissue. This is the case in rheumatic fever, where antibodies produced in response to a streptococcal infection attack the joints of the infected person. Other common autoimmune diseases are systemic lupus erythematosus, rheumatoid arthritis, rheumatic heart disease, and glomerulonephritis.

Acquiring Antibodies

There are several ways in which antibodies may be acquired. These may be grouped according to whether the body of the host manufactures the antibodies itself, thus producing *active immunity*; or whether the host's body receives ready-made antibodies from an outside source, as in *passive immunity*.

Active Immunity. When a person contracts a communicable disease, in most cases the body will respond by manufacturing antibodies against the pathogen or disease agent. Substances such as pathogens and other foreign agents that stimulate the production of antibodies are referred to as *antigens*.

A second way the body may be actively involved in the manufacture of antibodies is for the person to receive a *vaccination*, the process by which a person is injected with a vaccine containing either a dead, attenuated, or weakened pathogen, or a toxoid. When these substances are introduced into the body, they stimulate the production of antibodies, without inducing a disease state.

The protection conferred on the host as a result of either of the two circumstances just described is usually lifelong in duration, and is called active immunity.

Passive Immunity. Passive immunity may be acquired (1) via an injection of a serum; (2) by the fetus through the placenta; and (3) by the baby while breast-feeding. In each case, the antibodies received by the host are produced somewhere other than in the host's body.

Acquiring Passive Immunity. (1) When a serum is injected into a person, it confers immediate protection on the recipient against whichever disease agent or pathogen the antibodies are designed to respond to. A *serum* is a substance that contains antibodies made by an animal that has been injected with a pathogen. In response to the pathogen, the animal produces antibodies which are subsequently withdrawn from its body, treated in a laboratory, and made into a serum.

(2) Beginning with the third month of pregnancy, antibodies from the mother pass through the placenta into the fetal circulation, thus providing temporary protection at birth to the baby from whichever diseases the mother had acquired antibodies against. This protection may last anywhere from one to six months after birth.

(3) In addition to the placental transfer, antibodies may be passed to the baby through breast milk. This strengthens the baby's ability to resist those diseases against which the mother has acquired antibodies.

Active Immunity vs. Passive Immunity. While each type of immunity protects against disease, one differs from the other in terms of how quickly protection is provided, and how long it will last. Active immunity requires approximately two to three weeks for antibodies to be developed; once developed, however, they usually last for the span of the host's life. On the other hand, passive immunity confers immediate, on-thespot protection, although it is relatively short-lived. Antibodies received through the injection of a serum may be effective for only two weeks, while those received through placental transfer and breast milk may last as long as six months.

In summary, the third-line defense represents the body's last and innermost barrier to disease. It consists of antibodies which are protein substances that must be acquired, and which respond only to the specific antigens that initially stimulated their production. Antibodies confer immunity: if they are manufactured within the host's body, the immunity is called active; if they are produced outside the host's body and then introduced, passive immunity is conferred on the host. Both varieties of immunity protect against disease. Active immunity is usually lifelong in duration, but requires several weeks to become effective. Passive immunity is relatively short-lived, but takes effect immediately.

Resistance and Levels of Prevention

The body's lines of defense work in concert to provide ongoing protection against disease. As such, their effectiveness becomes a measure of the host's level of resistance. In other words, according to the first biological law of disease, the body's lines of defense prevent the imbalance that results in disease.

Primary Prevention Level

Preventing this imbalance first occurs at the *primary prevention level*. Primary prevention may be defined as taking those steps to maintain one's resistance at as high a level as possible. With respect to the *individual*, primary prevention consists of all the practices subsumed under the heading of good personal hygiene. These include: keeping the body clean, getting adequate rest, having a balanced diet, exercising regularly, and getting regular checkups.

However, primary prevention efforts are not limited to the individual. The *community and government* must also take primary prevention steps to prevent this imbalance, such as providing a safe water supply; cleaning streets; removing garbage; disposing of wastes safely; passing laws governing food handling and preparation; inspecting eating places; setting standards for safety; educating the public about health matters; informing the public about health hazards; and addressing poverty and its concomitant problems of unemployment, homelessness, crime, and lack of health care.

Primary prevention refers to all of the steps taken *before* disease occurs. These steps are designed to enhance the ability of the lines of defense to work at maximal efficiency, thus maintaining resistance at the highest level possible.

Secondary Prevention Level

When primary prevention efforts fail to keep the host from falling ill, *secondary prevention* measures need to be taken. Secondary prevention refers to those actions taken once disease has set in; that is, *after the fact*. In general, these actions are designed to contain the disease, keep it from worsening, and when possible, rid the host of the disease. They include seeking medical intervention, and clearly following whatever medical advice is given; both are responsibilities of the individual. However, it is the responsibility of the community/government to insure access to medical intervention so that healing can take place and disease may be contained.

Tertiary Level of Prevention

A third level, *tertiary prevention*, comes into play when the host requires rehabilitation. These actions are designed to restore to the greatest extent possible those abilities or capacities that the host may have lost as a result of illness. At this level of prevention, the roles of the individual and community/government are identical to those at the secondary level.

With respect to the Biological Laws of Disease, it is clear that the individual and the community/government are partners in (1) preventing the imbalance that results in disease, (2) minimizing the impact of disease through early detection and treatment, and (3) maintaining as healthy and safe an environment as possible.

THE NATURAL HISTORY OF ANY DISEASE IN MAN

Chart 1.1, The Natural History of Any Disease in Man I, depicts the interrelationships between host, agent, and environment, as well as the three levels of prevention. It also provides some examples of how the roles of the individual and community/government need to mesh for a given level of prevention to be effective.

Chart 1.1 and Chart 1.2, The Natural History of Any Disease in Man II, are divided into two time frames: a *prepathogenesis* period and a *pathogenesis* period.

Prepathogenesis

The prepathogenesis period is the time *before* disease actually develops. As shown in Chart 1.2, it is that phase of the disease cycle when host and agent come together and a disease state may develop. At this point, the effectiveness of the body's lines of defense becomes apparent. If they succeed in repelling the invading agent, and/or preventing its lodging in the body, the host will remain in a prepathogenic state. However, if the lines of defense are not able to do this, the agent will lodge and multiply. This stage in the natural history of a communicable disease is known as the *incubation period*.

Chart 1.1
The Natural History of Any Disease in Man I

PREPATHOGENESIS PERIOD	PATHOGENESIS PERIOD	
Primary Prevention Measures	**Secondary Prevention Measures**	**Tertiary Prevention Measures**
<u>By the Individual:</u> Good personal hygiene Acquiring effective coping skills Regular check-ups etc.	<u>By the Individual:</u> Seeking professional care Complying with professional advice etc.	<u>By the Individual:</u> Seeking professional advice Complying with professional advice etc.
<u>By the Community/Government:</u> Addressing the problem of poverty and its related problems Ensuring access to health care Protection from environmental hazards Prevention of accidents	<u>By the Community/Government:</u> Ensuring access to health care Case finding measures Screening surveys etc.	<u>By the Community/Government:</u> Ensuring access to care Providing hospitals and facilities for rehabilitation, limiting disability, and preventing death, etc.

Source: Adapted from a chart distributed to an epidemiology class at Columbia University School of Public Health, 1965.

Chart 1.2
The Natural History of Any Disease in Man II

The Course of the Disease In Man

Interrelations of the various

AGENT

HOST

and

ENVIRONMENTAL FACTORS

which bring AGENT and HOST together

and which may produce a disease state

in the Host

Recovery
PREPATHOGENESIS PERIOD

CLINICAL HORIZON --------------------

Tissue and physiologic
changes

AGENT becomes established
and multiplies and spreads

PATHOGENESIS PERIOD

Death
Chronic State
Disability
Illness

Signs and Symptoms

Resistance
and
Immunity

Source: Adapted from a chart distributed to an epidemiology class at Columbia University
School of Public Health, 1965.

Incubation Period

During this stage, the pathogen is growing and multiplying in preparation for its disease-producing mission. The incubation period may be considered the crossover point between prepathogenesis and pathogenesis.

Pathogenesis

The pathogenesis period occurs *after* the lines of defense have been breached. Initially, the interaction of host and agent may produce no discernible signs or symptoms.

Signs and Symptoms. *Sign* of disease is defined as an *objective* indicator or measure of disease; for example, a fever, tumor, rash, bleeding, or elevated blood pressure. These are phenomena that can be measured, seen, or felt. On the other hand, *symptom*, means a *subjective* response to illness, which cannot be measured. Symptoms include feelings or sensations such as pain, fatigue, and weakness.

In early pathogenesis, neither signs nor symptoms may be present. However, as pathogenesis progresses, various tissue and physiologic changes begin to take place, and signs and symptoms finally do appear. These not only alert the host that something is wrong, but also enable the physician to make a diagnosis and prescribe a course of treatment.

The *clinical horizon* is an imaginary line which separates pathogenesis into two phases: (1) *below* the clinical horizon, when no signs or symptoms appear; and (2) *above* the clinical horizon, when they do. Being below the clinical horizon does not mean that no disease activities are taking place, only that the disease has not yet progressed far enough for signs and symptoms to show. Above the clinical horizon, the progression of the disease is indicated, along with possible outcomes: recovery, disability, or death. Implicit in this progression is the efficacy of the body's lines of defense, the physician's diagnosis and treatment protocol, and the host's degree of adherence and response to the treatment.

DISEASE-RELATED TERMINOLOGY

When used in a disease context, some common terms have a meaning that differs from their everyday usage. Because they are basic to the understanding of disease, it is important to define them.

Incidence and *prevalence* are two examples of such terms. When used in a disease context, incidence refers to the number of *new* cases of a disease occurring since a certain date. For instance, one might say that since July 1 of this year, the incidence of tuberculosis was twelve. Prevalence always refers to the *total number* of cases of a disease that are in existence at a given time, so one might say that as of July 1 of this year, there were "x" number of cases of tuberculosis. Prevalence includes both new and old cases of a disease.

Endemic, epidemic, and pandemic are also frequently used to describe diseases. *Endemic* means that a disease is usually present in a given geographic area, such as malaria is endemic to many tropical locations. *Epidemic* means that the number of new cases of a disease exceeds the expected incidence of that disease for a certain area. Hence, even one or two cases could be considered an epidemic for an area where a specific disease had not previously occurred. Expected incidence is based on records of disease occurrence. It is a well established fact, for example, that January and February are peak incidence months for influenza in the northeastern part of the United States. Should July have an incidence rate for influenza equal to that of January or February, a state of epidemic would be declared. *Pandemic* means that a disease is worldwide, not limited to one geographic area. AIDS is an example of such a disease.

Morbidity rate refers to the number of cases of a disease at a stated time in relation to the population of an area. It is expressed as a fraction, with the number of disease cases as the numerator and the population as the denominator. Similarly, *mortality rate* indicates the number of deaths at a stated time in relation to the population. It, too, is expressed as a fraction, with the numerator being the number of deaths and the denominator the population. The population may include all of the people in an area at a given time, or it may be limited to a specific age group, ethnic group, or sex, depending on what sort of relationship is being studied.

Incubation period is the time span between the entrance of the pathogen or germ into the body and the appearance of signs and symptoms.

Period of communicability refers to the time during which a disease may be spread from one source to another.

SUMMARY

The Biological Laws of Disease, the body's lines of defense, and the natural history of any disease comprise a framework for understanding the disease process. Each of these aspects of disease development explains when and how a disease may take hold in the host, and what the possible outcomes of such an occurrence might be. Also, they delineate the roles of the individual and the community/government in prevention, detection, containment, and management of disease.

This framework is applicable to both communicable and non-communicable diseases. In the case of a communicable disease, the causative agent is always a pathogen, or germ. In non-communicable disease, the term *risk factor* or *precipitating factor* should be substituted for *causative agent*. The term *host* always refers to the recipient of the causative agent, or the person affected by the risk or precipitating factor. Resistance refers to the host's ability to ward off the causative agent in communicable disease, or the effects of the risk factor in non-communicable disease. The term *environment* always refers to external conditions which may impact the host.

LEARNING OBJECTIVES

From the information included in this chapter, the student will be able to:

1. write the three Biological Laws of Disease.
2. tell how each law relates to communicable and non-communicable diseases.
3. define the terms *host, agent,* and *environment* with respect to the Biological Laws.
4. tell what is meant by the nature and characteristics of the agent.
5. define the terms that relate to agent characteristics.
6. tell what comprises each of the body's lines of defense.
7. describe how each line of defense functions.
8. identify two ways in which active immunity may be acquired.
9. identify three ways in which passive immunity may be acquired.
10. define the term *antigen.*
11. distinguish between the three levels of prevention.
12. identify the two phases of the natural history of a disease.
13. explain the significance of the clinical horizon.
14. define the terms *endemic, epidemic, pandemic, prevalence, incidence, morbidity,* and *mortality.*

REFERENCES

Benenson, A. S., ed. *Control of Communicable Disease Manual.* 16th ed. Washington, DC: American Public Health Association, 1996.

Campbell, J. "Making Sense of Immunity and Immunization." *Nursing Times* 90: 32–34, 1994.

Crowley, L. V. *Introduction to Human Disease.* 4th ed. Boston: Jones and Bartlett, 1996.

Edelson, P. J. "Editorial: The Need for Innovation in Immunization." *AJPH* 85: 1613, 1995.

Fairbrother, G., and K. A. DuMont. "New York City's Child Immunization Day: Planning, Costs, and Results." *AJPH* 85: 1662–65, 1995.

Guyton, A. C., and J. E. Hall. *Textbook of Medical Physiology.* 9th ed. Philadelphia: W. B. Saunders, 1995.

Krieger, N. "Analyzing Socioeconomic Patterns in Health and Health Care." *AJPH* 83: 1086–87, 1993.

Lewy, R. *Preventive Primary Medicine*. Boston: Little, Brown, 1980.

Purtilo, D. T., and R. B. Purtilo. *A Survey of Human Diseases*. 2nd ed. Boston: Little, Brown, 1989.

Sheldon, H. *Boyd's Introduction to the Study of Disease*. Philadelphia: Lea and Febiger, 1984.

Smith, D. T., N. F. Conant, and J. R. Overman. *Zinnser Microbiology*. 13th ed. New York: Appleton-Century-Crofts, 1964.

Timmreck, T. C. *An Introduction to Epidemiology*. Boston: Jones and Bartlett, 1994.

2

COMMUNICABLE
DISEASES

COMMUNICABLE DISEASE DEFINED

Four criteria must be met for a disease to be classified as *communicable*: (1) the presence of a host, (2) the presence of a disease-producing agent, (3) a mode of transmission, and (4) a mode of entry.

The *host* is the person who encounters the disease-producing agent, and who becomes *susceptible* when his or her lines of defense are unable to prevent the entrance, lodging, multiplication, and spread of that agent. In other words, a susceptible host is a person whose resistance is unable to fight off the invading pathogen.

Pathogen Characteristics

The disease-producing agent is known as a *pathogen*. Pathogens have four characteristics: virulence, infectivity, pathogenicity, and antigenicity. *Virulence* refers to the strength or power of the pathogen to produce disease. *Infectivity* is the ability of the pathogen to lodge or gain a foothold in the body, representing the first step in the disease-producing process. *Pathogenicity* refers to the pathogen's ability to multiply and spread; further steps in the disease-producing process. *Antigenicity* is the ability of the pathogen to stimulate the production of antibodies. These four characteristics describe the interaction of pathogen and host.

Reservoir refers to the site where the pathogen lives, and on which it depends for survival. Examples of reservoirs are: a human host, an animal, insects, soil, and water. To state this another way, the reservoir may be considered the source of contamination, as in the case of soil and water; or the carrier of the pathogen, as in the case of man, animals, and insects.

Classification of Pathogens

Pathogens that affect man may be classified as (1) bacteria, (2) rickettsia, (3) viruses, (4) fungi, (5) protozoa, (6) helminths, and (7) arthropods.

Bacteria are one-celled plant-like organisms that occur in three different shapes: a ball or sphere, called *coccus*; a rod, called *bacillus*; and a spiral, called *spirochete*. There are several varieties of cocci. For example, the *staphylococcus* causes food poisoning and styes of the eyes; the *streptococcus*, which is responsible for such diseases as streptococcal sore throat, scarlet fever, and streptococcal pneumonia; the *gonococcus*, which is responsible for gonorrhea; and the *meningococcus* which causes meningitis. *Bacilli* are responsible for such diseases as diphtheria, tuberculosis, botulism, salmonellosis, and cholera. Syphilis and lyme disease are caused by the *spirochete* variety. Figure 2.1 illustrates the three types of bacteria.

Rickettsia are disease organisms closely related morphologically to bacteria. Unlike bacteria, however, they require an insect vector to complete the disease transmission cycle. Therefore, rickettsia cause diseases in which a tick, flea, or body louse acts as the intermediary between the host (man) and the animal reservoir on which it was living, and from which it obtained the rickettsia. Typhus fever, Rocky Mountain spotted fever, and Q fever are three examples of diseases caused by rickettsia.

Viruses are the smallest of all the pathogenic organisms that attack man. They are *parasitic*, requiring a living host in order to survive, and have the quality of *tropism*, which is the ability to attach themselves to receptors on the surface of living cells. The presence or absence of a receptor on a given cell determines whether that cell will become infected. From this vantage point on the receptor, the virus can release enzymes which enable it to penetrate the cell. Once within the cell, the virus has the ability to multiply and spread, thus creating a disease state. However, it may also merely enter the cell and remain

Figure 2.1
Three Types of Bacteria. (A) Cocci, (B) Bacilli, (C) Spirochete.

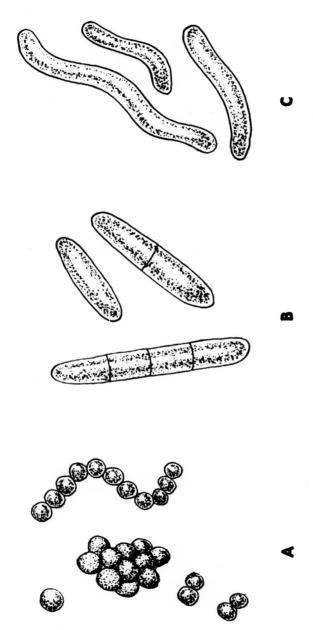

Source: Health For Better Living by M. Hurster. Englewood Cliffs, N.J.: Prentice-Hall, Inc., 1964, p. 240.

there without altering or interfering with the cell's normal functioning.

One way of classifying viruses is to name them according to the tissue they infect. For example, *neurotropic*—focusing on the nervous system and causing such diseases as poliomyelitis, rabies, and encephalitis; *dermotropic*—those which cause smallpox, rubella, measles, mononucleosis, herpes simplex, and herpes zoster; *pneumotropic*—responsible for the common cold, viral pneumonia, mumps, influenza, and conjunctivitis; and *viscerotropic*—those which cause yellow fever and the various strains of hepatitis.

Fungi are single- or multicelled plants which lack chlorophyll and are generally characterized as molds or yeasts. Many, but not all, forms of fungi are pathogenic to man. The diseases they produce are known collectively as *mycoses*. Superficial mycoses include ringworm and athlete's foot. Deep-seated mycoses, also called systemic mycoses, include infections of the mucous membranes and lungs, such as moniliasis.

Protozoa are one-celled, microscopic animals that are parasitic in nature and exist in either an active stage, called *trophozoite*, or in an inactive stage, called *cyst*. It is during the trophozoite stage that the protozoa create an infection in the host. In the cyst stage, the protozoa lodge in the host's body without creating a disease state, and the host becomes a carrier and potential transmitter of the protozoa to another host.

There are two main groups of protozoa: the intestinal, oral, and genital protozoa; and the blood and tissue protozoa. The first group causes such diseases as amebiasis and giardiasis. Malaria is the best known disease caused by the second group of protozoa.

Helminths are parasitic worms. It has been estimated that almost a third of the earth's human inhabitants harbor some kind of parasitic worm. Three main groupings of helminths exist: roundworms, tapeworms, and flukes. Once they enter the body, they lodge in the intestines and/or tissues, and go through their life cycle there. Life cycle stages consist of: the unfertilized egg, the egg, the larva, and adulthood. Some helminths are infective in the egg stage, others in the larva stage. Infestation of the host does not always initially produce observable signs of disease. Nevertheless, the helminth is robbing the host of food, and may be releasing harmful toxins into the host's body, causing damage. In time, the effects of infestation will become apparent. Weight loss; swelling of the legs, scrotum, and breasts; anemia; and muscular pain are some of the clinical manifestations of worm infestation. Hookworm disease, ascariasis, trichinosis, beef tapeworm, and pork tapeworm are some diseases caused by helminths. Figure 2.2 illustrates some of the helminths that infest man.

Arthropods are parasites which live on the surface of the host's body. Lice, fleas, ticks, and mites are the principal arthropods that affect man. They may play either a direct or indirect role in the causation of disease. Their role is considered *direct* when they create skin eruptions or introduce poisonous venom into the body. When they serve as the vector, or carrier, in disease transmission, their role is considered *indirect*. Pediculosis, or head lice, is an example of direct causation, and Lyme disease may be described as indirect.

Mode of Transmission

This term refers to the way a communicable disease may be spread from one source to another. Transmission may occur between people, between man and animals, and between man and plants. There are three modes of transmission: (1) inhalation, (2) contact, and (3) ingestion.

Inhalation is the taking in of air and droplets or particles carried by the air. Pathogens that are transmitted this way include representatives from the viral, bacterial, and fungi groups.

Contact is the coming together of the host with an infected

Figure 2.2
Four Types of Helminths. (A) Tapeworm, (B) Roundworm, (C) Trichina, (D) Liver Fluke.

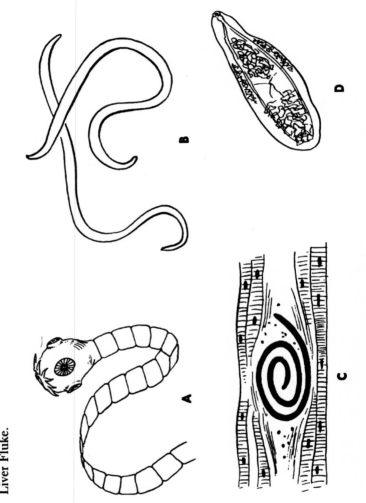

Source: *Health For Better Living* by M. Hurster. Englewood Cliffs, N.J.: Prentice-Hall, Inc., 1964, p. 240.

person, insect or animal, or a contaminated object and/or environment. Representatives from all the pathogen groups are capable of being transmitted in this manner.

Ingestion is the swallowing of food and drink containing disease-producing organisms. Helminths and bacteria are the types of pathogens spread in this manner.

Mode of Entry

This term refers to the portal or opening through which the pathogen gains entrance to the body. For those diseases transmitted through the air, the portal is the nose or mouth. In diseases spread via contact, the portal is the skin and/or mucous membranes lining such body orifices as the vagina, anus, and mouth. For diseases spread via ingestion, the entryway is the mouth and digestive tract.

CATEGORIES OF COMMUNICABLE DISEASES

Communicable diseases may be categorized according to their mode of transmission; a given disease having several modes of transmission may belong to more than one category. For example, many of the childhood diseases may be spread via inhalation in addition to direct contact.

Respiratory refers to diseases that are spread via inhalation. These include measles, chicken pox, mumps, rubella, tuberculosis, the common cold, and influenza.

Integumentary diseases are spread via contact and include AIDS, STDs, rabies, Lyme disease, conjunctivitis, and hepatitis B.

Alimentary is the name for diseases spread via ingestion. Included in this category are hepatitis A, typhoid fever, cholera, and trichinosis.

RELATIONSHIP OF EACH DISEASE GROUP
TO FRAMEWORK

Respiratory Group

Prepathogenesis. During this stage of the disease process, host, agent, and environment interact with each other. In respiratory diseases, host and agent are brought together via the inhalation of airborne particles, some of which may be pathogenic.

The environment may serve as a transmission enabler in a number of ways. For example, an environmental factor such as crowding could increase the likelihood of spread. Similarly, exposure to cold inhibits the flow of blood to the surface and orifices of the body, thus reducing the number of leukocytes available to combat potential sources of infection. As host and agent come into contact with each other, the first-line defenses come into play, especially the cilia and mucous membranes. The cilia are designed to filter out foreign particles; however, if they have become coated with tars as a result of smoking, or flattened from exposure to such environmental hazards as asbestos or lead, their filtering ability is diminished, and their effectiveness as a line of defense lessened.

The mucous membranes provide a sticky surface to which foreign particles may adhere, thus halting their further penetration of the respiratory system. Their ability to do this, however, is limited by their surface area. Hence, if they are exposed to large numbers of particles, it may not be possible to contain all of them, and some will penetrate the breathing passages, thereby breaching the first-line defenses.

Pathogenesis. In early pathogenesis, the pathogen is most likely to initially settle in the nose, throat, or sinuses. Coughing, sneezing, running nose, fever, and sinus headache will probably accompany this stage of the disease process. The appearance of these signs means that the disease has moved above the clinical horizon. It now becomes the role of the second-line defenses to contain the pathogen and prevent its spread to other parts of the respiratory system. As pathogenesis progresses, the lymph glands may become swollen as a result of destruction of pathogenic organisms by lymphocytes, and the white blood cell count will probably be elevated. Antibodies (the third line of defense), produced as a result of the infection, will also attempt to halt it from spreading further. Should these responses fail to curb the infection, the pathogen will continue to move more deeply into the respiratory system, ultimately settling in the lungs and producing a full-fledged case of disease. From this point on, the host will either recover from the disease or succumb to it.

If the host recovers, it is likely that he or she will have built up an immunity against future encounters with this particular pathogen. It is also possible that the host may become a carrier of the pathogen. Chart 2.1, The Natural History of Chicken Pox, is a depiction of the disease process just described.

Integumentary

Prepathogenesis. For this group of diseases, prepathogenesis is comprised of interactions between the host, an agent, the environment, and in some cases, a vector or fomite. The skin and mucous membranes, which line all body orifices, are the portals of entry for these diseases. A *vector* is an insect or animal that passes the disease agent to the host. A *fomite* is an inanimate object that transmits the agent to the host. The environment plays a significant role in the transmission of these diseases insofar as it provides suitable breeding places for vectors, such as flies and other insects. A warm, moist environment is suitable for the growth of fungi, such as may be found after bathing, between the toes and body folds, or when one is overheated. Mucous membranes, which are also warm and moist, may serve as potential breeding sites for various pathogens.

Integumentary diseases are spread via *direct contact* with the

Chart 2.1
The Natural History of Chicken Pox

PREPATHOGENESIS

——virus enters host via either direct contact or inhalation of droplets

——body's first-line defenses fail to repel the virus and it lodges in nose, throat, and eyes initially

——once a lodging place is found, virus proceeds to multiply and become infective

PATHOGENESIS

——as virus becomes infective, the body's second-line defenses (white blood cells and lymphocytes) come into play

——virus is carried to lymph nodes for elimination; as a result, lymph nodes become enlarged and white blood cell count is elevated indicating the presence of infection

——second-line defenses fail to halt the spread of the virus; it invades the liver and spleen

——————————————— CLINICAL HORIZON ———————————————

——virus moves to skin, causing chicken pox rash to develop

——as rash begins to disappear and disease to subside, the virus enters nerve endings and lodges there in a dormant state

RECOVERY

POSSIBLE SEQUELAE

——if the host's level of resistance is weakened later on in life, the virus can return to an active state and bring on an episode of shingles, a painful nerve inflammation source of infection, through a *break in the skin* caused by an insect or animal bite, or a cut caused by an unsterile object. For example, conjunctivitis may be spread by touching discharge from the eyes of an infected person and then touching one's own eyes, or by using a tissue or eye-drop dispenser previously used by an infected person. Hepatitis B, AIDS, and sexually transmitted diseases (STDs) may be transmitted via sexual intercourse, during which direct contact with the exudates of lesions or infected tissue may take place. In Lyme disease, the transmission involves an interaction between the host, an agent, a vector, and the environment.

Pathogenesis. Once the integrity of the skin is broken, as in the case of an insect or animal bite, or via a cut or wound from an unsterile object, pathogens gain direct entrance into the underlying tissue and blood circulation of the host, thereby beginning the pathogenesis stage of disease development. When this occurs, the area surrounding the break in the skin may become inflamed. The inflammation is marked by swelling, redness, heat, and pain. These signs represent the body's initial efforts to resist the invading pathogens, and their presence indicates that the disease has moved above the clinical horizon. Following the onset of inflammation, pus may develop at the site of the break. Pus is comprised of dead pathogens and leukocytes, and is a sign that the second-line defenses have become activated. If these early-defense responses fail to halt the pathogen's spread, a full-fledged case of the disease is likely to develop, and the host will pass through the subsequent stages of pathogenesis.

Rabies is an example of a disease that is transmitted via the bite of an infected animal. Lyme disease is spread through the bite of a tick. Hepatitis B and AIDS may be spread via unsterile hypodermic needles and dental picks, as well as through the transfusion of blood products such as plasma or platelets that have not been screened for these diseases.

Another way in which hepatitis B and AIDS may be spread is from an infected pregnant woman to her fetus through the placenta. While this mode of transmission does not fit the break-in-the-skin category, the seriousness and widespread nature of these diseases necessitate its mentioning. Tetanus may result from stepping on a rusty nail while barefoot, or a cut from an unsterile knife.

The other mode of transmission for integumentary diseases is via direct contact with the source of infection. When the pathogen comes into contact with either the skin or the mucous membranes lining a body orifice, it attempts to attach itself to that surface and establish a lodging place where it can grow and multiply. If the surface of the skin is unclean or moist, it becomes a desirable lodging place for fungi. Diseases transmitted in this way include athlete's foot and the various forms of ringworm. They are marked by a scaly, itchy outbreak on the surface of the body which, if untreated, has the tendency to spread to adjacent tissue.

If the pathogen attacks the mucous membranes, a lesion or sore usually develops at the initial point of contact between the pathogen and the membrane. The area around the sore or lesion becomes inflamed, a pussy discharge may develop, and pain may be experienced. This is the course that is followed in many of the STDs, with the exception of syphilis and gonorrhea. In syphilis, a sore (known as a chancre) will appear at the point of contact between pathogen and membrane. The chancre is neither painful nor accompanied by inflammation, and will disappear in four to six weeks, with or without treatment. In gonorrhea, no lesion or sore develops; instead, the membrane becomes inflamed and discharges a yellowish pus. Inflammation will spread, causing ulceration of the membrane and adjoining tissue, ultimately interfering with the tissue's functioning.

Once this first line of defense has been breached, the pathogen will try to gain a foothold in the host's body, multiply, and spread. As it is doing this, the second and third-line defenses will attempt to thwart its growth and development. During this period, signs and symptoms of disease will appear, and the disease stage is considered to be above the clinical horizon. From this point on, the host will pass through the various stages of pathogenesis, and will either recover from the disease, or die from it.

Alimentary

Prepathogenesis. Diseases belonging to this group are spread through the food and drink that we swallow, initiating the prepathogenesis stage. Pathogens causing alimentary diseases attempt to either invade the mucous membrane lining the digestive tract, thereby leading to ulceration and acute inflammation of the membrane, or produce toxins which interfere with normal metabolism. Hepatitis A, typhoid fever, salmonellosis and trichinosis are examples of diseases in this group.

Pathogenesis. This stage begins when the body attempts to rid itself of the pathogen by means of vomiting or diarrhea. These reflex acts comprise the first-line defenses against this group of diseases. Nausea, fever, and chills usually accompany the vomiting and diarrhea, and abdominal cramps may also be experienced. In most cases, the first-line defenses will not succeed in halting the infection, and the second- and third-line defenses will be called into play. Signs and symptoms resulting from their intervention may include an elevated leukocyte count, and jaundice in the case of hepatitis A. Once the second- and third-line defenses are involved, pathogenesis will progress through its various stages, and the host will either recover (with or without adverse residual effects) or succumb to the disease.

SUMMARY

Communicable diseases can be spread from one source to another, either through the air we breathe, a break in the skin, direct contact with a pathogen, or through the food and drink we swallow. Diseases spread through the air are known as respiratory diseases, through a break in the skin or via contact are

Figure 2.3
Breaking the Chain of Infection

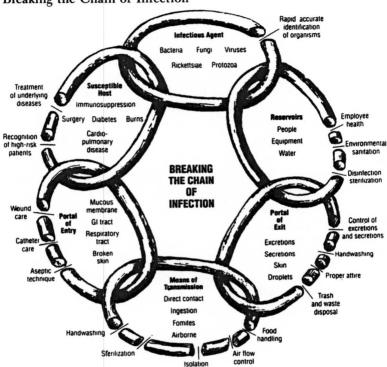

integumentary diseases, and through food and drink are called alimentary diseases. Figure 2.3, Breaking the Chain of Infection, illustrates these methods of transmission.

No matter how a communicable disease is spread, it always involves a host (man) and a causative agent (a pathogen, or germ). Pathogens that attack man are classified as: bacteria, rickettsia, viruses, fungi, protozoa, helminths, and arthropods. To varying degrees, all pathogens possess the characteristics of virulence, infectivity, pathogenicity, and antigenicity.

All communicable diseases pass through two stages: (1) a

prepathogenesis stage, in which host, causative agent, and environment interact, and when the body's first-line defenses attempt to prevent the pathogen from gaining a foothold in the host's body; and (2) a pathogenesis stage, in which the second and third lines of defense are called on to fight off the invading pathogen once it has succeeded in getting past the first line of defense. Signs and symptoms will appear during the pathogenesis stage. The conclusion of pathogenesis is marked by either the host's recovery or death. Recovery may or may not be accompanied by disability.

LEARNING OBJECTIVES

From the information included in this chapter, the student will be able to:

1. list the four criteria of a communicable disease.
2. name the three groups of communicable diseases, as well as their modes of transmission and entry.
3. give an example of a disease in each group.
4. describe the prepathogenesis and pathogenesis stages of each group.
5. identify the seven groups of disease-producing organisms in man.
6. give an example of a disease caused by each group of organisms.

REFERENCES

Benenson, A. S., ed. *Control of Communicable Disease Manual.* 16th ed. Washington, DC: American Public Health Association, 1996.
Bickley, H. C. *Practical Concepts in Human Disease.* 2d ed. Baltimore: Williams and Wilkins, 1977.
Brooks, S. M. *Basic Facts of Medical Microbiology.* Philadelphia: W. B. Saunders Company, 1962.
Crowley, L. V. *Introduction to Human Disease.* 4th ed. Boston: Jones and Bartlett, 1996.

Evans, A. S., and P. S. Brachman. *Bacterial Infections of Humans: Epidemiology and Control*. 2d ed. New York: Plenum Medical Book Co., 1991.

Mandell, G. L., R. G. Douglas, Jr., and J. E. Bennett, eds. *Principles and Practices of Infectious Diseases*. 3d ed. New York: Churchill Livingstone, 1992.

Timmreck, T. C. *An Introduction to Epidemiology*. Boston: Jones & Bartlett, 1994.

3

NON-COMMUNICABLE DISEASES

Non-communicable diseases as a group account for more than 70% of all deaths in the United States today; ranking first, second, and third as cause of death. Because most of them are incurable and require lifelong management and control, their toll on health care costs is astronomic. Therefore, it is no wonder that the principal focus of *Healthy People 2000*, a U.S.P.H.S. statement of health goals for the American public, should be the reduction in incidence of this group of diseases.

NON-COMMUNICABLE DISEASE CRITERIA

All diseases which do not fit the basic criteria of a communicable disease are designated as non-communicable. That is, they are not caused by a pathogen, and cannot be spread via airborne droplets, ingestion of contaminated food and drink, or direct contact from the host to another person.

Definition

In non-communicable disease, some part or parts of the body cease to function as they were intended. In other words, a non-communicable disease occurs when a body part or parts become either *nonfunctioning* or *malfunctioning*. Often, but not always, this is incurable and lifelong in duration, requiring ongoing treatment or management to prevent the host's demise and/or further incapacitation.

Precipitating or Risk Factors

The malfunctioning or nonfunctioning may be related to the *host's genetic makeup,* such as sex, race, or a family history of a disease like diabetes, heart disease, or cancer. It may also develop as a consequence of some aspect of the *host's lifestyle,* such as diet, a lack of or too much exercise, inability to cope with stress, smoking, or drug-taking. It may be a natural concomitant of the *aging process*; result from exposure to such *environmental hazards* as radiation, air pollution, or noise; or it may be due to such *social factors* as homelessness, unemployment, or poverty. All of these factors which have the potential to bring about the malfunctioning or nonfunctioning of a body part are known collectively as *precipitating* or *risk factors*. The greater the number of risk factors impacting the host at a given time, the greater the likelihood that he or she will develop a non-communicable disease.

RELATIONSHIP OF NON-COMMUNICABLE DISEASES TO THE DISEASE FRAMEWORK

Prepathogenesis

When relating the disease framework to non-communicable diseases, several adjustments need to be made. First, the term *precipitating factor* or *risk factor* should be substituted for *agent*. Second, the environment should be subsumed under the risk factor heading. Hence, for non-communicable diseases, prepathogenesis begins when the host interacts with or is impacted by precipitating or risk factors. This interaction may or may not lead to a disease state. The genetic makeup of the host, the number and strength of the risk factors impacting him or her at a given time, and the duration of their impact determine whether a state of pathogenesis will ensue.

Pathogenesis

Unlike most communicable diseases, the development of a non-communicable disease is insidious. It comes about in small increments, which initially may be passed off by the host as too inconsequential to merit professional attention. Vague feelings of fatigue, weakness, and occasional spasms of pain are examples of signs that the host may overlook, and yet may presage the pathogenesis stage of a non-communicable disease.

It is important to note that it may take a considerable length of time for a fully developed disease state to appear. Examples include the development of lung cancer in smokers only after years of smoking, and the onset of osteoarthritis in athletes years after their retirement from active competition. Educating the public as to the warning signs of non-communicable diseases is an important first step in detection, which, in turn, is an important factor in minimizing the impact of the disease on the host. This means slowing down or halting the progression of pathogenesis. To do this, appropriate interventions need to be employed. Successful intervention requires cooperation between the host and his or her care giver. This presupposes that the host has a care giver. Therefore, even though informing the public about warning signs, possible interventions, and sources of care are necessary steps in the control and management of non-communicable diseases, unless *access to care* is provided, these steps will be ineffective, and the ultimate consequences of unrestrained pathogenesis will occur; namely, incapacitation and/or death.

GROUPS OF NON-COMMUNICABLE DISEASES

Genetic

A person's genetic makeup is determined at the *moment of conception*, when sperm and egg unite. The characteristics conferred at this time are designated as *inherited characteristics*, and are determined by the *genes* carried by the two sex cells. Genes, in turn, are situated on *chromosomes*. Every cell of the human body contains twenty-three pairs of chromosomes, or forty-six in all. Inherited characteristics are immutable and include (but are not limited to): hair, skin, and eye color; sex; potential body shape and size; potential for intellectual, artistic, musical, athletic, or mechanical achievement; and the potential for developing such diseases as hypertension, diabetes, cancer, Alzheimer's disease, and Tay-Sachs disease, as well as the actual development of such genetic disorders as hemophilia, muscular dystrophy, sickle-cell disease, phenylketonuria, and Down's syndrome. Genetic disorders may result from chromosomal abnormalities and mutations, which may have been induced by exposure to radiation, environmental chemicals, and maternal infections. A brief description of these diseases and disorders is provided at the end of this chapter.

Inherited, Congenital, and Acquired Characteristics. It is important to differentiate between *inherited* characteristics, which are *gene-based*, and those that develop in-utero; that is, after conception but before birth. These are known as *congenital* characteristics, which do not have a genetic base. Their onset may be attributed to a variety of causes that for the most part are related to the behavior of the pregnant woman. These include: inadequate diet and/or prenatal care; consumption of drugs and alcohol; smoking; trauma resulting from a fall or blow to the abdominal region; excessive exposure to an environmental hazard; and being infected with AIDS, syphilis, gonorrhea, or rubella. Examples of problems that may develop in-utero include: mental retardation, AIDS, fetal alcohol syndrome, cleft palate, spina bifida, congenital herpes simplex, congenital syphilis, congenital rubella, and a variety of organ and limb abnormalities. With good prenatal care, some of these problems can be prevented. One of the most frequently occurring problems for the fetus is being born prematurely.

Prematurity. Being *born prematurely*, or *prematurity*, is defined as weighing less than 2,500 grams, or 5½ pounds, at birth. A low birthweight means that the fetus's vital organs are not yet fully developed, thus minimizing its chances of survival. Other possible effects on the fetus are that it may be born either without a body part, or without an intact or correctly functioning body part. Prematurity may also result in a shortened life span and mental retardation.

Educating about pregnancy, the importance of prenatal care throughout the pregnancy, and providing access to prenatal care are functions of society's health care delivery system. As a nation, we have not been particularly effective in performing these functions. Globally, the United States, which spends more on health care than any other nation, ranks twenty-first in infant mortality and tenth in maternal mortality. Moreover, according to Kotelchuck's "Adequacy of Prenatal Care Utilization Index," one in six American women has inadequate prenatal care, and almost two in five have less than adequate care. These data identify an aspect of the American health care delivery system that requires more attention and support.

A third group of characteristics that differs from both inherited and congenital is that of *acquired characteristics*. These develop either as the baby is exiting the womb, or at any time after delivery, and they are not gene-based. Included in this grouping are problems that may arise during the birth process, as well as the many health problems that all of us are subject to during our lives.

Problems that may arise during the birth process include: (1) the baby presenting itself buttocks-first instead of headfirst, thus necessitating a breech delivery; (2) the umbilical cord may become wrapped around the baby, cutting off his or her air supply; and (3) infections of the cervix may be passed on to the baby during delivery.

Prenatal Testing. It is now possible to identify the genetic makeup of a person. In the case of pregnancy, we may predict with considerable accuracy the appearance of a genetic defect in the child being carried. When the pregnancy has advanced to approximately the fifteenth week, this prediction can be verified through *amniocentesis*, a surgical procedure in which a sample of amniotic fluid (the fluid in which the baby is immersed during pregnancy) is withdrawn and examined for the presence of abnormal chromosomes. *Ultrasound scanning* is another procedure that can be used to determine whether the fetus is developing normally. This involves using high-frequency sound waves which are reflected off the fetus, converted into pictures, and displayed on a screen. These pictures can reveal the presence of multiple fetuses, fetal head size, and abnormal brain development. A third detection method is *chorionic villus analysis*, which is a diagnostic technique for early detection of genetic abnormalities. It involves inserting a thin tube into the uterus and removing a small sample of chorionic material and examining it for abnormal chromosomes.

Chorionic villi are outgrowths of the chorion, the outer layer of the amniotic sac which surrounds the fetus during pregnancy. They attach themselves to the endometrium, the lining of the uterus, and serve as exchange stations for oxygen, nutrients, and wastes between mother and fetus. They comprise part of the placenta. This test can be performed as early as the eighth week of pregnancy.

Should the results of any of these detection methods reveal the presence of a defect, the parents would be faced with the difficult decision of whether to carry the pregnancy to term or abort. It is their physician's responsibility to clearly explain the consequences of either decision. Prior to pregnancy, genetic testing and counseling can alert a couple to the fact that one or both of them may be carrying defective genes and/or chromosomes. Regardless of whether these tests are performed before or after conception, the decision of how to proceed will fall to the woman and her partner. It is imperative that their decision be based on fact.

Heart-Related Diseases

These are diseases involving the heart, as well as the blood vessels both within and outside the heart. They may be genetic in origin, the consequence of life-style factors, aging, exposure to environmental hazards, or due to various social factors. One of the interesting and unfortunate features of this group of diseases is that the onset of one of them almost always leads to the development of another. For example, a condition of atherosclerosis (in which the arteries become clogged with plaque) will likely lead to elevated blood pressure. In turn, elevated blood pressure, or hypertension, may lead to coronary heart disease, cerebrovascular disease, or both. And all may result in death. Therefore, it is important to keep in mind that heart-related diseases share common causes, and have a cause-and-effect relationship with each other. Before discussing this group of diseases, an explanation of the heart, as well as its role in circulation and other parts of the circulatory system, is necessary.

Structure of the Heart. The heart is a muscular organ about the size of an adult's clenched fist, and is situated in the chest region. Its function is to pump blood around the body—which it performs throughout a person's life. Along with the blood vessels and blood, it comprises the body's circulatory system.

The heart is made up of four chambers: two upper receiving chambers, known as *atria* or *auricles*; and two lower discharging chambers, known as *ventricles*. The atria and ventricles are separated by walls containing *valves*, which regulate the flow of blood between them. The *tricuspid valve*, located between the right atrium and ventricle, remains shut while the atrium is filling with blood. When it is completely filled, sensors in the wall of the atrium signal the valve to open, allowing the blood to pass into the ventricle. The *bicuspid* or *mitral valve* performs a similar function on the left side of the heart. A cross section of the heart is shown in Figure 3.1.

Heart Murmur. To insure maximum output of blood per heart contraction, it is essential that the valves work efficiently; that is, they should not leak. When valves do not close completely, blood seeps into the ventricle, resulting in a less than maximal output of blood by the heart. This condition is known as *heart murmur*. People with heart murmurs tire easily, experience shortness of breath upon the slightest exertion, and may develop an enlarged heart.

The heart is divided lengthwise by a wall, known as the *septum*, which prevents blood from passing from one side to the other. This is an important function because the blood that passes through the right side of the heart is deoxygenated. It has a lower oxygen content, as well as a high concentration of

Figure 3.1
Cross Section of Heart

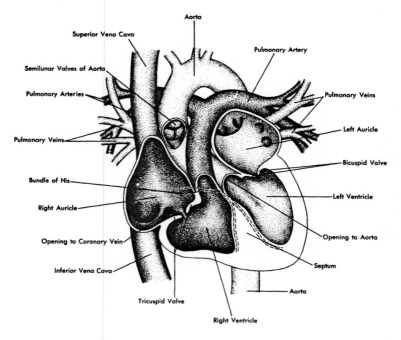

Source: *Health For Better Living* by M. Hurster. Englewood Cliffs, N.J.: Prentice-Hall, Inc., 1964, p. 181.

carbon dioxide, a waste product given off by all body cells. This
blood must first be sent to the lungs for reoxygenation and
removal of carbon dioxide before passing through the left side
of the heart and then on to the rest of the body. Babies born
with an opening in the septum are known as *blue babies*. The
bluish cast to their skin is due to the oxygen deprivation they
are experiencing because of the recirculation of deoxygenated
blood.

Path of Blood Through the Heart. Deoxygenated blood
(that has been collected from all the cells of the body) enters
the right atrium via the two largest veins in the body: the

superior and inferior vena cava. The superior vena cava brings this blood from the upper part of the body; the inferior vena cava brings it from the lower part of the body.

The deoxygenated blood passes from the atrium, through the tricuspid valve, and into the right ventricle. From there it is carried by the *pulmonary artery* to the lungs, where the carbon dioxide is removed and oxygen replaced. This process is called *diffusion.* Diffusion may be further defined as the passage of substances through a semipermeable membrane *from* an area of denser concentration *to* an area of lesser concentration. Thus, when the deoxygenated blood with its high concentration of carbon dioxide and low concentration of oxygen reaches the lungs, carbon dioxide diffuses into the *alveoli* (air sacs) of the lungs, and oxygen diffuses from the alveoli into the blood. In this way, the blood is cleansed of its waste products and reoxygenated. This newly oxygenated blood is then transported back to the heart by the *pulmonary vein,* which connects with the left atrium. The oxygenated blood passes through the left atrium, through the bicuspid valve, and into the left ventricle, then exits the heart via the aorta, the largest artery in the body. The aorta separates into many smaller arteries which carry the oxygenated blood to all the cells of the body. This pathway of blood through the heart is shown in Figure 3.2.

Heart rate, the rate at which the heart contracts, is regulated by several masses of nerve tissue situated within the heart: the *sinoatrial node,* or *pacemaker,* located in the right atrium; *the atrioventricular node,* located in the ventricles; and the *Bundle of His,* also found in the ventricles. Figure 3.3 shows their location in the heart. The sinoatrial node sets the rate of contraction, which is then transmitted to the other nerve masses, and via them to the rest of the heart. Although the heart has its own intrinsic way of maintaining the rate of beat, it can be altered by impulses arising from the nervous system during times of stress, exposure to excessive heat, physical exertion, and illness. The average normal heart rate, or pulse rate, for

Figure 3.2
Flow of Deoxygenated Blood Through the Body

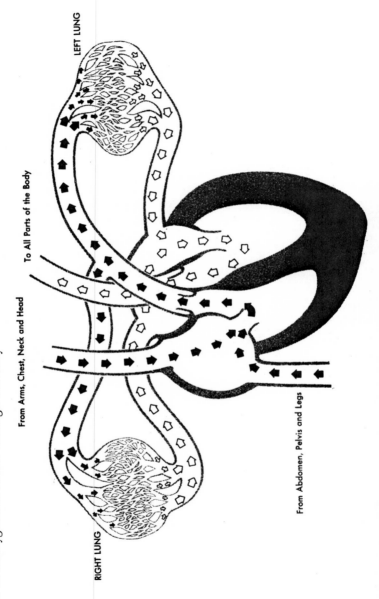

LEFT LUNG

To All Parts of the Body

From Arms, Chest, Neck and Head

RIGHT LUNG

From Abdomen, Pelvis and Legs

Source: Health For Better Living by M. Hurster. Englewood Cliffs, N.J.: Prentice-Hall, Inc., 1964, p. 183.

Figure 3.3
Location of Heart Nodes

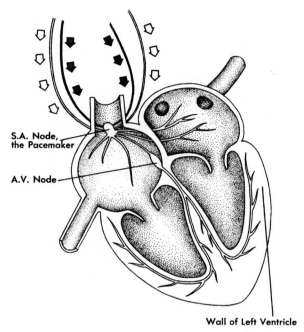

Source: *Health For Better Living* by M. Hurster. Englewood Cliffs, N.J.: Prentice-Hall, Inc., 1964, p. 182.

an adult while sitting is approximately seventy-two beats per minute. This rate is higher when standing and during exercise, and lower when lying down.

Blood Pressure. In contrast to how *fast* the heart is beating at any given time, is the degree of *force* exerted by the heart as it pumps blood, called *blood pressure*. There are two measurable blood pressures in the body: systolic and diastolic. *Systolic pressure* is a measure of the *force* with which the heart must contract in order to empty the ventricles of blood. *Diastolic pressure* is a measure of *arterial resistance* to the volume of blood being pumped out by the heart. Blood pressure is

Chart 3.1
Classification of Blood Pressure for Adults

Category	Systolic (mm Hg)	Diastolic (mm Hg)
Normal	<130	<85
High normal	130–139	85–89
Hypertension		
Stage 1 (Mild)	140–159	90–99
Stage 2 (Moderate)	160–179	100–109
Stage 3 (Severe)	180–209	110–119
Stage 4 (Very Severe)	≥210	≥120

Source: Clinician's Handbook of Preventive Services. U.S. Dept. of Health and Human Services. Public Health Service, 1994, p. 137.

measured by a sphygmomanometer, and expressed in terms of millimeters (mm) of mercury (Hg). For an adult, a normal systolic pressure reading is 120 mm Hg, and a normal diastolic reading is 80 mm Hg. The upper limits of normal pressure are 140 mm Hg over 90 mm Hg. When readings exceed these, a condition of *high blood pressure*, or *hypertension*, is said to exist. Chart 3.1 gives the classification of blood pressure levels for adults.

The Blood Vessels. There are three kinds of blood vessels in the body: arteries, veins, and capillaries. *Arteries* always carry blood *away* from the heart. They complement the pumping action of the heart by contracting in concert with it. Their walls are thick, muscular, and elastic, enabling them to push blood around the body. As the heart contracts, the arteries open, or dilate, to admit the volume of blood being pushed out. Then, as the heart relaxes, the arteries contract, moving the blood further along the circulatory system. As an artery subdivides, it gets smaller and smaller; the smallest of which are known as *arterioles* and possess the same properties as arteries.

Veins always carry blood *toward* the heart. Their walls contain valves, or cups, which catch and hold the blood between heart contractions, enabling them to move blood upward toward the heart against the pull of gravity, thus keeping it from flowing downward toward the feet. Veins also subdivide; small veins are known as *venules* and have the same properties as larger veins.

Capillaries are the smallest blood vessels in the body, and serve as the exchange stations for oxygen, nutrients, and wastes between the blood and the cells. It is through their one-cell-thick walls that diffusion takes place. In each cell of the body there is a network of arterioles, venules, and capillaries, with the capillaries linking the smallest arterioles and venules. Figure 3.4 illustrates the three types of blood vessels and their functional relationship.

Blood is the body's transport system for delivery of nutrients and oxygen to the cells, and removal of waste products from the cells. It is made up of plasma, red blood cells, white blood cells, and platelets.

Plasma is the liquid portion of the blood, comprising three-fifths of its total volume. It consists mostly of water, contains a large amount of protein material, acts as the transport system for red cells, white cells, and platelets, and is the medium in which diffusion takes place.

Red blood cells, or *erythrocytes,* primarily transport oxygen and carbon dioxide. They synthesize and carry hemoglobin, a compound made from protein and iron, which enables them to perform these functions. Red blood cells are manufactured by the bone marrow. Up to puberty almost all of the bones perform this function. From puberty to approximately age twenty the long bones gradually cease doing this, and the task falls to the vertebrae, ribs, and sternum. As a person ages, the rate at which these bones produce red cells decreases, so that by old age it is likely he or she will be slightly anemic.

White blood cells, or *leukocytes,* are formed in both bone

Figure 3.4
Three Types of Blood Vessels

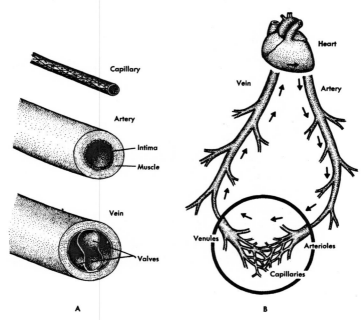

Source: Health For Better Living by M. Hurster. Englewood Cliffs, N.J.: Prentice-Hall, Inc., 1964, p. 185.

marrow and the lymph nodes. Their role is to ingest foreign matter that has infiltrated the body's lines of defense.

Platelets are the clotting elements of the blood that keep us from bleeding to death when we are injured. They contain a variety of proteins which form clots when tissue is damaged and bleeding ensues. In the inherited disease hemophilia, one or more of the proteins needed for clotting is missing.

Some Important Heart-Related Diseases

Hypertension. Approximately one in every four Americans suffers from *high blood pressure*, or *hypertension*. In general, elevated blood pressure results when there is a *constriction*, or *closing*, of the blood vessels, especially of the arteries, and/or when deposits accumulate on the inner walls, or intima, of the arteries. In both cases, the flow of blood through the heart and circulatory system is impeded, and this interference forces the heart to work harder to move blood around the body.

Constriction of blood vessels is the body's natural response to a *stimulant*. Thus, when we smoke, the nicotine (which is classified as a stimulant) causes constriction of blood vessels and temporarily elevates blood pressure. The caffeine in coffee, tea, and cola drinks has a similar effect. Certain widely used amphetamines, such as benzedrine, dexedrine, and ritalin act as stimulants, and some illicit drugs also produce this effect.

In addition to those occasions when we *deliberately* use one of the aforementioned substances, constriction of blood vessels occurs when the adrenal gland releases *adrenaline* or *epinephrine*, a hormone which prepares the body to take action. This happens whenever we feel threatened; that is, whenever our safety or self-esteem is being challenged. The threat may be physical, as in the case of being confronted by a mugger; or related to our mental/emotional state, as in having to sit for an important exam or perform in front of an audience. It could also be due to a denigrating remark that someone has made about us.

Blood flow can also be impeded by *deposits* that have accumulated on the inner walls, or intima, of the arteries. These deposits are most frequently comprised of *cholesterol* and are called *plaque*. Cholesterol is a fatty substance manufactured by the body, and although it is a natural ingredient of the body, it becomes a problem when too much of it is produced. This may happen when the diet contains large quantities of foods that are rich in saturated fats, such as egg yolks, liver, red meats, butter, and whole milk.

As plaque is laid down on the intima, the opening within the artery for blood to pass through becomes smaller, making the heart contract with more force as it tries to move blood through the artery. As a result, blood pressure rises. When the body is *regularly* subjected to a diet rich in unsaturated fats and to the arterial constriction brought on by stimulants, it is easy to understand how a condition of hypertension may arise.

There are two types of hypertension: essential and secondary. *Essential* is the more common of the two, occurring in about 90% of all hypertension cases. It has no identifiable single cause, and no signs to alert a person that he or she might be harboring a serious health problem. For this reason, essential hypertension has been called "the silent killer." Its precipitating factors are well known, including: heredity; life-style factors, such as diet, smoking, and lack of regular exercise; aging; failure to effectively cope with stress; and such social factors as poverty, homelessness, and unemployment. African Americans have a higher incidence than other racial groups, and women have a higher incidence than men. People living under conditions of prolonged stress are also prone to essential hypertension. *Secondary hypertension*, on the other hand, occurs in a very small segment of the population, usually resulting from either kidney disease or an endocrine abnormality, such as excessive thyroid gland activity or a disorder of the adrenal glands.

When blood pressure remains elevated over time, various parts of the body become damaged. Most susceptible to damage by prolonged hypertension are the heart, eyes, brain, and kidneys. One of the first effects on the *heart* is that it will become enlarged in an attempt to compensate for the increased resistance to blood flow. In time, this attempt will fail, first resulting in lowered efficiency of heart function, and eventually in failure.

Another effect of prolonged hypertension is the breaking down of capillaries within the heart. This results in hemorrhaging of blood, which interferes with the functioning of the heart, and eventually leads to heart failure. When capillaries hemorrhage in other organs, their function is also interfered with, leading to serious consequences. Thus, hemorrhaging in the eyes may result in blindness; in the brain, paralysis or even death; and in the kidneys, further elevation of blood pressure, toxemia, and possibly death.

To avoid and/or break this chain of consequences, several steps need to be taken. First, the host must have his or her blood pressure taken to ascertain whether he or she is hypertensive. If the reading is high normal, or high, the host would be advised to follow a physician's recommendations for dealing with the problem. These may include: limiting the intake of saturated fats, losing weight, increasing physical activity, and quitting smoking. If the reading indicates that hypertension already exists, medication may also be prescribed. Lifelong vigilance and observance of these steps are essential in curbing the natural progression of this disease.

Atherosclerosis. This is a condition in which fatty deposits accumulate on the inner walls of the arteries. Behaviors that might bring on atherosclerosis include: a diet rich in saturated fats; physical inactivity; smoking, and obesity—all of which are modifiable. Since atherosclerosis is one of the major precursors of hypertension, it is advisable that the host make those behavior changes to either prevent the onset of this condition or reverse it. If this is not done, the condition will worsen, and the consequences of hypertension will ensue.

Arteriosclerosis. This condition arises when the walls of the arteries become less elastic, impeding the flow of blood and resulting in elevated blood pressure. This loss of elasticity is a natural concomitant of the aging process, but it can also be exacerbated by smoking and prolonged exposure to stress. When the host has both arteriosclerosis and atherosclerosis, he or she is a strong candidate for a stroke or heart attack.

Stroke. Also known as *cerebrovascular disease*, stroke is the third leading cause of death in the United States. This condition may arise either when a *clot lodges in a blood vessel in the brain* and occludes the flow of blood to that part of the brain, or when an *artery in the brain ruptures*, releasing blood into the tissue.

When a blood vessel in the brain is occluded, brain cells are deprived of oxygen and nutrients, and cease to function. As a result, the part(s) of the body they control also stop functioning. Sometimes the clot(s) responsible for this condition become dislodged, allowing blood flow through the area to be resumed, and the condition is reversed with little or no aftereffects. This can happen without any medical intervention; however, when dislodging does not occur, it is imperative that medication be prescribed to dissolve the clot. The shorter the period of blockage, the less likely permanent damage will result. Hence, it is essential that this condition be responded to quickly.

When a blood vessel in the brain ruptures, an intracerebral hemorrhage occurs, making it impossible for the affected part of the brain to function. Paralysis is the usual manifestation of stroke, regardless of the cause.

Coronary Heart Disease. This is the leading cause of death in the United States today. It is also called *ischemic heart disease* or *coronary artery disease.* Atherosclerosis is its main precursor. Occlusion of coronary arteries due to cholesterol deposits on the intima deprives that part of the heart of oxygen and nutrients, renders it incapable of functioning, and if the blockage persists, eventually leads to its demise. The progression of steps leading to coronary heart disease is similar to that preceding a stroke. The most common outcomes of this disease are myocardial infarction (heart attack), angina pectoris (chest pain), and sudden death.

Myocardial Infarction. This heart condition, also known as *heart attack,* occurs when the blood flow to the heart muscle, or myocardium, is abruptly cut off. This is usually due to the lodging of a clot in the coronary circulation, or hemorrhaging from a ruptured coronary blood vessel. Chart 3.2, Risk Factors of Heart-Related Diseases, summarizes the risk factors for each of the aforementioned diseases.

The clots responsible for these diseases (atherosclerosis, coronary heart disease, cerebrovascular disease, and myocardial infarction) consist of clumps of cholesterol that have broken

Chart 3.2
Risk Factors of Heart-Related Diseases

DISEASE	RISK FACTORS						
	Family History	Aging	Smoking	Lifestyle Inactivity	Lifestyle Diet	Obesity	Stress
Arteriosclerosis	•	•	•		•	•	•
Atherosclerosis	•			•	•	•	
Hypertension	•	•	•	•	•	•	•
Coronary Heart Disease	•	•	•	•	•	•	•
Cerebrovascular Disease	•	•	•	•	•	•	•
Myocardial Infarction	•	•	•	•	•	•	•

away from deposits which line the inner arterial walls. This breaking away results from the movement of blood through the artery. A moving clot is called an *embolus*; a lodged, stationary clot is a *thrombus*. Clots move via the blood circulation and have the ability to lodge anywhere in the body. Regardless of where they lodge, their effect is the same—interference with the flow of blood, and ultimately, the ability of the affected body part to function. It is essential that steps to dissolve the clot be taken as soon as possible.

A common affliction of people who stand on their feet for

most of the day is *phlebitis*. This condition arises when a clot lodges in a blood vessel in the leg, causing pain, tenderness, redness, and swelling. While phlebitis is not life-threatening, it is incapacitating, and may have serious economic effects if the affected person is no longer able to hold a job.

Chronic Respiratory Diseases

These are diseases related to the respiratory system, which is responsible for bringing air into, and expelling carbon dioxide from the body. The prepathogenesis stage for this group of diseases usually involves the interaction of the host with a variety of environmental factors. Pathogenesis develops as a result of prolonged exposure to those factors, and is exacerbated when genetic elements in the host predispose him or her to the disease.

The Respiratory System. This system consists of: the body openings through which air enters, i.e., the nose and mouth; the trachea, or windpipe; the bronchi, or bronchial tubes; bronchioles; and air sacs, or alveoli. The *nose* is lined with *mucous membrane* and *cilia*, which work as filters. Mucous membrane has a sticky surface to which dust and foreign matter adhere, and the cilia are tiny hairs in the nostrils which wave back and forth, sweeping out debris from the inhaled air.

The *trachea*, or *windpipe*, is situated in the throat area, and is the link between the head and chest for the passage of inhaled air. It, too, is lined with mucous membrane and cilia. In the chest region, the trachea branches into the *two bronchi*, which enter the lungs. The bronchi are also lined with mucous membrane and serve as passageways for air within the lungs. Each bronchus subdivides into smaller and smaller branches, called *bronchioles*. The smallest bronchioles connect with the *air sacs*, or *alveoli*, which are minute, grape-like structures that link up with capillaries and serve as the exchange points for oxygen and carbon dioxide.

The bronchi, bronchioles, and alveoli are parts of the respiratory system located within the lungs, and the nose, mouth, and trachea are located outside the lungs.

Path of Air Through the Body. Inspired or inhaled air, 21% of which is oxygen, enters the body either through the nose or mouth, passes through the trachea on its way to the bronchi, then to the bronchioles and alveoli. From the alveoli it diffuses through the capillary walls into the blood circulation. Figure 3.5 illustrates this pathway, through which oxygen reaches the blood. Expired or exhaled air follows exactly the same path, only in reverse order.

Inhalation and Exhalation. These processes are performed by the rhythmic expansion and contraction of the chest cavity and lungs. The *expansion* phase is produced when the diaphragm pulls down on the rib cage, as the external intercostal muscles pull out on it. These actions increase the size of the chest cavity and decrease the pressure within it to below that of atmospheric pressure. When this happens, air is drawn into the body. In the *contraction* phase, the internal intercostal muscles and the abdominal muscles cause the chest cavity to contract, resulting in exhalation of air. Figure 3.6 shows the action of the muscles involved in exhalation and inhalation.

Some Important Chronic Respiratory Diseases

Pulmonary Emphysema. This is one of the *chronic obstructive pulmonary diseases* (COPD), a group of disorders in which the flow of blood through the airways is obstructed. In emphysema, the airways principally affected are the alveoli; their walls become distended, or stretched, and lose elasticity. As these changes develop, the ability of the alveoli to serve as exchange points for oxygen and carbon dioxide is compromised, and the host will have difficulty breathing. As he or she strains to take in air, the alveoli may be ruptured. Long-term cigarette smoking is the primary risk factor in the prepathogenesis of this disease; however, the precise way in which cigarette smoke brings on emphysema is not altogether under-

Figure 3.5
Pathway of Air Through the Respiratory System

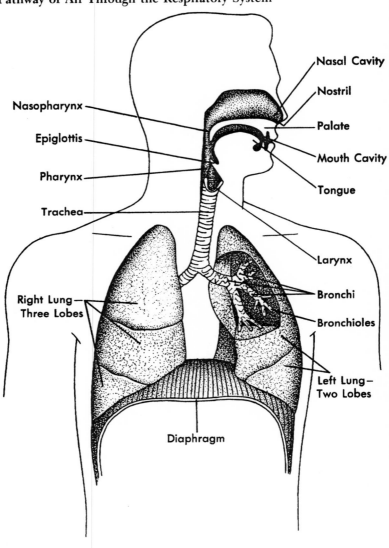

Source: Health For Better Living by M. Hurster. Englewood Cliffs, N.J.: Prentice-Hall, Inc., 1964, p. 176.

Figure 3.6
Muscles of Respiration

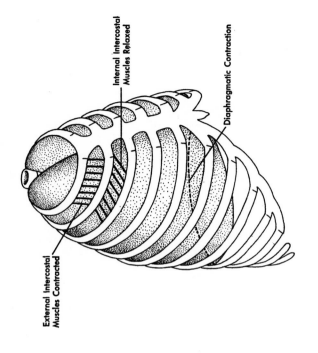

Internal Intercostal
Muscles Relaxed

External Intercostal
Muscles Contracted

Diaphragmatic Contraction

INHALATION

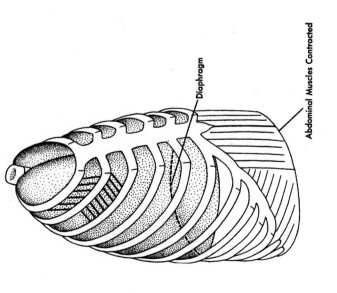

Diaphragm

Abdominal Muscles Contracted

EXHALATION

Source: *Health For Better Living* by M. Hurster. Englewood Cliffs, N.J.: Prentice-Hall, Inc., 1964, p. 177.

65

stood. Prolonged exposure to polluted air can also induce this condition.

In the pathogenesis stage of emphysema, the host first experiences shortness of breath upon exertion, and as the condition worsens, it is accompanied by wheezing and eventually heart failure. In general, emphysema is not reversible, but its progress can be slowed by not smoking and avoiding sources of air pollution.

Chronic Bronchitis. This disease is another of the COPD group; the airways obstructed in this case are the bronchi. Exposure to environmental agents, especially cigarette smoke, is the major precursor of this condition. For the host, its manifestations and consequences will be the same as for emphysema.

Asthma. Approximately 4% of the United States population is afflicted with this disease; children under eighteen and adults over seventy-five account for the bulk of these cases, the distribution of which is similar for males and females, but almost half again as high for African Americans as for whites. Whether this is due to a genetic factor, namely race, or an environmental factor, namely stress, is a matter of conjecture.

Asthma is a disease in which the airways become obstructed with mucus. Swelling, or edema, of the mucous membranes which line the airways may also bring on an asthmatic episode. Asthma may be classified as *allergic* or *nonallergic* in origin. People with allergic asthma can be identified through a battery of skin tests for common allergens. Those with nonallergic asthma will not respond to these tests. However, many asthmatics suffer from both varieties, and exhibit the same signs and symptoms.

Chronic Occupational Lung Diseases. Most of these diseases result from the inhalation of dust particles, and are named for the agent associated with them, including: asbestosis (asbestos); silicosis (silica); byssinosis (cotton dust); and black lung disease, or coal miner's pneumoconiosis (coal dust). In the prepathogenesis stage, the host encounters the dust particles, with prolonged exposure leading to pathogenesis. Exposure to multiple agents, as in the case of a host who is also a cigarette smoker, will hasten the onset of disease.

Cancer

This is the second leading cause of death in the United States today, with an annual incidence of almost 1.2 million cases. Cancer is a *progressive condition* in which there is *uncontrolled growth and spread of abnormal cells* occurring anywhere in the body. Lung cancer is the most frequently occurring form of this disease.

Cancers may be categorized according to histologic or anatomic site. There are five major *histologic* categories of cancers: (1) *carcinomas*, found in the surface cells of the skin, breasts, lungs, urinary, reproductive, and gastrointestinal tracts, and glands of the body; (2) *melanomas*, found in the melanin-producing cells of the skin, placenta, ovaries, and testes; (3) *lymphomas*, found in the lymph nodes, spleen, and thymus gland, and generally classified as Hodgkin's disease; (4) *leukemias*, found in the bone marrow; and (5) *sarcomas*, found in connective tissue, bone, fat, blood vessels, lymph vessels, and smooth and striated muscle tissue. Carcinomas account for 80–90% of all cancers; lymphomas for approximately 5%; leukemias about 4%; sarcomas about 2%, and melanomas for less than 1%.

The five most prevalent anatomic sites of cancer are: the lungs, colon/rectum, breasts, prostate gland, and uterus. These are categorized by incidence and death rate in Chart 3.3.

Prepathogenesis. The initial development of cancer is precipitated by exposure to a *carcinogen*, or cancer-inducing factor. Carcinogens take many forms, including: the tars in tobacco smoke; excessive radiation from both the environment and laboratory procedures; and environmental hazards, such as asbestos, vinyl chloride, and benzene. Since cancer seems to run in families, it is likely that there is an *inherited predispo-*

Chart 3.3
Common Cancer Sites

Rank	Cancer Incidence		Cancer Deaths	
	Male	Female	Male	Female
1	Prostate 200,000	Breast 182,000	Lung 94,000	Lung 59,000
2	Lung 100,000	Colon/Rectum 74,000	Prostate 38,000	Breast 46,000
3	Colon/Rectum 75,000	Lung 72,000	Colon/Rectum 27,800	Colon/Rectum 28,200
4	Bladder 38,000	Uterus 46,000	Pancreas 12,400	Ovary 13,600
5	Lymphoma 29,400	Ovary 24,000	Lymphoma 12,100	Pancreas 13,500
6	Oral 19,800	Lymphoma 23,500	Leukemia 10,500	Lymphoma 10,650
7	Melanoma 17,000	Melanoma 15,000	Stomach 8,400	Uterus 10,500
8	Kidney 17,000	Pancreas 14,000	Esophagus 7,800	Leukemia 8,600
9	Leukemia 16,200	Bladder 13,200	Liver 7,200	Liver 6,000
10	Stomach 15,000	Leukemia 12,400	Bladder 7,000	Brain 5,800
11	Pancreas 13,000	Kidney 10,600	Brain 6,800	Stomach 5,600
12	Larynx 9,800	Oral 9,800	Kidney 6,800	Multiple Myeloma 4,800
All Sites	632,000	576,000	283,000	255,000

Source: Clinician's Handbook of Preventive Services. U.S. Dept. of Health and Human Services. Public Health Service, 1994, p. 148.

sition to its development. Clearly, it is very important for the person with a family history of cancer to minimize exposure to carcinogens.

Pathogenesis. Cancer begins when the DNA of a normal cell is mutated by a carcinogen, resulting in a cell that is quite different. This mutated cell grows and multiplies at a much faster rate than normal cells, resulting in a cell colony which fails to perform normal functions and also interferes with the normal cells by usurping their space and food supply. Consequently, the normal cells die, and the part of the body that they comprise eventually loses its ability to function.

Malignant and Benign Tumors. Cancer cells form colonies, or masses, known as *malignant tumors*; growths which have the ability to spread. Other growths, such as *benign tumors*, do not have this capacity. While both kinds of tumors may disrupt a body function, malignant tumors are far more serious. Figure 3.7 depicts the difference in appearance between these two types of tumors.

Metastasis is the term used to describe the spread of cancer cells from one site to another. Once cancer cells have metastasized, it is all but impossible to completely rid the body of them. Therefore, early detection is of the utmost importance.

Detection Measures. To enable the public to detect cancer early, the American Cancer Society has formulated a list of common warning signs. These include: a change in the size or appearance of a mole or wart; persistent sore throat, indigestion, or hoarseness; a thickening or lump; a sore that does not heal; unexplained change in bowel or bladder functions; unexplained bleeding or discharge from a body opening; and persistent cough. Appearance of any of these signs does *not* mean that cancer is present; however, the opinion of a physician should be sought as quickly as possible to determine their significance.

In addition to publishing this list of warning signs, a concerted effort has been made to encourage women to practice breast self-examination, and men to practice testicular self-

Figure 3.7
Cross Section of Benign and Malignant Tumors

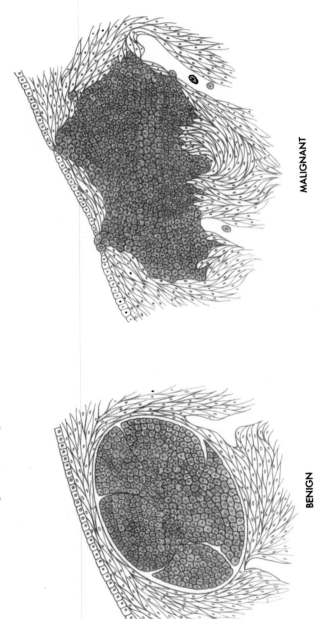

BENIGN

MALIGNANT

Source: Health For Better Living by M. Hurster. Englewood Cliffs, N.J.: Prentice-Hall, Inc., 1964, p. 278.

examination. In addition, women between the ages of forty and forty-nine have been advised to have a mammogram every one to two years, and annually after fifty years of age.

The *clinical determination of cancer* is usually accomplished by a *biopsy*, a procedure in which cells are taken from the affected site and examined by a pathologist. Since cancer cells differ markedly in appearance from normal cells, they are quite easy to detect.

Stages of Cancer. Cancers are classified according to the extent of tumor spread. *Stage 0* is defined as a precancerous state, in which cancer cells are *in situ*, but have not yet burrowed into, or invaded, the tissue on which they are situated. People with this stage need to be closely monitored for signs that the cancer has become invasive.

Stage 1 cancers are localized and premetastatic. The cancer cells have begun to infiltrate the tissue on which they are situated, but have not yet spread to other sites in the body. To prevent further infiltration and metastasis, surgical removal of the cancer is indicated when possible. If the location of the cancer precludes the use of surgery, radiation therapy should be promptly employed.

Stage 2 are cancers in which further infiltration of underlying tissue has taken place, but they are still considered to be premetastatic. Immediate removal of the cancer should be implemented to prevent further spread. Surgery and radiation are indicated as treatment modalities.

Stage 3 are cancers in which metastasis has occurred, and there is involvement of adjacent tissue and organs. Surgery, radiation, and chemotherapy are indicated as appropriate treatment modalities.

Stage 4 cancers are advanced cases of the disease in which there has been extensive spread throughout the body. Little can be done at this stage other than to make the patient as comfortable as possible.

Common Cancer Sites. Although no part of the body is immune to cancer, some parts tend to be affected more often than others. In females, the seven most frequently affected sites listed in descending order include: the breasts; lungs; colon and rectum; uterus; ovaries; lymphatic system; and the skin. For males, these include: the prostate; lungs; colon and rectum; bladder; mouth; skin; and kidneys.

Treatment for Cancer. This includes surgery, radiation, and chemotherapy. *Surgery* involves excising the tumor. This treatment modality is most effective when utilized before metastasis has occurred. To make certain that all cancer cells in the vicinity of the excision have been destroyed, radiation of the area is employed as a complementary procedure. When the tumor is inaccessible; that is, when its location prohibits the use of surgery due to the possibility of damaging a vital body part, other treatment modalities are resorted to.

Radiation will destroy cancer cells; however, it also has the potential to destroy normal cells and can produce reactions that may range from acute to chronic. Acute reactions usually appear soon after the treatment and subside within a few weeks or months. They include: extreme sensitivity of the irradiated skin to sun, heat, and tight clothing; recurring nausea; abdominal cramps; the need to urinate frequently; diarrhea; and hair loss. More serious and, in some cases, long-lasting responses to radiation include: a lowered sperm count and sterility in men if the genitalia have been radiated; and termination of ovarian hormone production in women, which may lead to temporary or permanent menopause.

Radiation is usually administered via three techniques: external beam; implantation of a sealed, radioactive source; and systematic administration of a radioisotope. The *external beam technique* involves aiming a beam of X rays or gamma rays at the targeted area. In general, a series of such treatments is necessary, and may be performed on an outpatient basis. In the second technique, a *sealed, radioactive source* is implanted in the affected tissue and left there for a few days; this may also be performed on an outpatient basis. *Systematic administration of a radioisotope* usually requires hospitalization of the patient until all the radioactive material has dissipated.

Chemotherapy involves the administration of chemical agents for the purpose of destroying cancer cells, thus halting the disease's progression. They are usually administered intramuscularly, and travel through the body via the bloodstream to the cancer site(s). While they are effective in destroying cancer cells, they also harm normal cells, and are responsible for numerous unpleasant side effects. Hair loss, nausea, and diarrhea are some of the less serious of these; more serious effects include destruction of white blood cells and platelets. Since white blood cells are needed to ward off infections, their destruction reduces the body's ability to resist disease. Platelets play a prime role in blood clotting, and loss of them results in hemorrhaging. Therefore, patients receiving chemotherapy need to be carefully monitored for these conditions.

Immunotherapy is another treatment modality in which chemical agents are administered. In this case, however, their purpose is to augment the body's immune system rather than destroy cancer cells.

Endocrine-Related Diseases

The endocrine glands serve as *regulators* of various vital bodily functions. They do this by secreting chemical substances, called *hormones*, directly into the blood. Each hormone is programmed to control or regulate a specific part of the body. The *principal endocrine glands* include: the hypothalamus; thyroid; parathyroids; pituitary; adrenals; the islets of Langerhans in the pancreas; and the gonads, i.e., testes and ovaries.

The *hypothalamus* is part of the brain stem. Its principal hormone is *thyrotrophin*, which stimulates the production of thyrotrophic hormone by the anterior pituitary gland. This hormone is responsible for enlargement of the thyroid gland when production of thyroxin falls below acceptable levels. Enlargement of the thyroid is also known as goiter.

The *thyroid gland* is situated in the neck region below the larynx. Its principal hormone is *thyroxin*, which regulates the basal metabolic rate of the body.

The *parathyroids* are found in the neck region behind the thyroid gland. These four glands regulate calcium and phosphorus metabolism, as well as vitamin D utilization in the formation of bones and teeth. Their principal hormone is *parathormone*, or *parathyroid hormone*.

The *pituitary gland* is located at the base of the brain. It consists of two parts: the *anterior pituitary*, or *adenohypophysis*; and the *posterior pituitary*, or *neurohypophysis*.

The anterior pituitary releases a number of hormones. The *growth hormone* stimulates growth in body tissues. *Corticotropin*, also known as *ACTH*, acts on the adrenals in the metabolism of carbohydrates, fats, and proteins. The *follicle-stimulating hormone* plays a role in the production of estrogen by the ovaries. *Luteinizing hormone* regulates the ovulation function of the ovaries, and the production of testosterone by the testes. *Luteotrophic hormone* regulates the production of progesterone and estrogen during the ovarian cycle, and breast milk following pregnancy.

The posterior pituitary's principal hormones are *antidiuretic hormone* and *oxytocin*. Antidiuretic hormone regulates the concentration level of body fluids. A lack, or underproduction, of this hormone is related to the onset of *diabetes insipidus*. Signs of this condition include extreme thirst, a strong desire for salty foods, and frequent, copious urination. Oxytocin acts on the female reproductive system and the anterior pituitary, initiating labor by causing the uterus to contract. Also, it stimulates the production of luteotrophic hormone by the anterior pituitary.

The *adrenal glands* are located near the kidneys. Each has two parts: an adrenal medulla and an adrenal cortex. The adrenal medulla produces two hormones which affect the nervous system: *epinephrine* and *norepinephrine*, which determine the "fight/flight" response. The adrenal cortex produces three hormones: *aldosterone*, *cortisone*, and *androgen*. Aldosterone is a mineralocorticoid, which regulates the level of concentration of sodium, potassium, and chlorides in body fluids. Cortisone is classified as a glucocorticoid, and plays important roles in suppressing inflammation, regulating the level of glucose concentration in the blood, and in metabolism of carbohydrates, fats, and proteins. Androgen promotes masculinization.

The *pancreas*, which contains the *islets of Langerhans*, is located near the abdomen. Insulin, its primary hormone, is responsible for glucose metabolism and mobilizing glycogen from the liver and skeletal muscles when the glucose concentration of the blood is lowered.

The *gonads*, or *sex glands*, are the ovaries in the female and the testes in the male. The *ovaries* produce ovarian hormones, known collectively as estrogens. These hormones cause the ovaries to achieve their full growth, and are also responsible for the appearance of the female secondary sex characteristics. These include: development of the breasts, growth of underarm and pubic hair, widening of the pelvis, and the onset of menstruation. Figure 3.8 illustrates the effects of the female sex hormones on the menstrual cycle.

The *testes* produce testosterone, which is responsible for the development of male secondary sex characteristics. These include: proliferation of underarm, pubic, and facial hair; production of sperm; broadening of the shoulders; toughening of the skin; lowering of the voice; and thickening of the musculature.

An *endocrine-related disease* develops when a gland either ceases to produce a sufficient quantity of a hormone, or produces too much of one. The prefix *hypo* is used to indicate an insufficient quantity, and *hyper* to suggest an overabundance. In either case, the regulatory function is disturbed, sometimes with a devastating effect on the host. Malfunctioning of an endocrine gland may be due to an inherited predisposition, or to a tumor or lesion.

Some Important Endocrine-Related Diseases

Diabetes Mellitus. More than 6.8 million people in the United States have been diagnosed as diabetic, and diabetes mellitus is now the country's seventh leading cause of death.

Figure 3.8
Menstrual Cycle Hormones

PHASE	GROWTH		OVULATION	SECRETORY		PREMENSTRUAL	MENSTRUATION
	Early	Advanced		Early	Advanced		
DAYS	4-8	9-13	14	15-18	19-25	26-28	1.3 to 5
CHANGES	1) growth of primary follicle and ovum 2) growth of new endometrium			1) ovum in tube 2) change of follicle into corpus luteum	1) secretions of estrogens and progesterone by corpus luteum 2) preparation of endometrium for pregnancy	Regression of endometrium begins due to degeneration of corpus luteum and withdrawal of estrogens and progesterone	
GONADO-TROPHIC HORMONES	FSH			Luteinizing	Luteotrophic		
OVARIAN HORMONES	Estrogens			Estrogen and Progesterone			None

Source: Health For Better Living by M. Hurster. Englewood Cliffs, N.J.: Prentice-Hall, Inc., 1964, p. 102.

This is a disease in which the body either fails to produce sufficient *insulin,* a hormone which regulates glucose metabolism, or to utilize the insulin it does produce. The islets of Langerhans cells in the pancreas are responsible for producing insulin. When they fail to do this, *glucose,* the body's primary source of energy, cannot be metabolized, is dumped into the blood, and ultimately into the urine. This causes the concentration of glucose in both these fluids to rise, so that by measuring it, diabetes may be detected.

When the body cannot metabolize glucose, it converts glycogen, adipose tissue, and even protein into energy because it must have an ongoing supply to continue functioning. Of these three sources, glycogen is the smallest but most efficacious. Degradation of adipose tissue and protein represents an inefficient and limited way of providing energy. Unless the problem of insulin production and/or utilization is addressed, the host will die.

Types of Diabetes. There are two major types of diabetes: Type I, or *insulin-dependent diabetes mellitus*; and Type II, *non-insulin-dependent diabetes mellitus.*

Type I was originally called juvenile diabetes because its onset usually occurs in childhood or adolescence. It is the less-frequently occurring of the two types, and requires lifelong administration of *injected* insulin. Type II was originally called adult-onset diabetes mellitus because it usually appears after age forty. Depending on the severity of the disease, it may be possible to control this type by means of diet and regular exercise. Oral administration of insulin is also indicated as a control modality.

Numerous risk factors are implicated in the prepathogenesis of both types of diabetes mellitus. A genetic predisposition appears to be common to each type; in Type II, the life-style factors of obesity and inactivity exacerbate this predisposition, and hasten the development of the disease.

As the disease progresses, signs and symptoms will appear. In Type I, there will be an *abrupt* appearance of such symptoms as excessive thirst, frequent urination, and weight loss. These same symptoms will also appear in Type II, but will do so gradually. The clinical signs for both types include elevated levels of glucose in the blood and urine, and accumulation of ketone bodies in the blood and body tissues. Ketone bodies result from the degradation of protein into energy, and create a condition of acidosis in the blood and body tissues, which, if uncorrected, will be lethal.

Thyroid Disorders. The thyroid gland, located in the throat region, produces the hormone *thyroxin*, which regulates the body's metabolic rate. Metabolism is the rate at which all cells of the body expend energy. Figure 3.9 illustrates the way in which food is metabolized.

Types of Thyroid Disorders. In *hyperthyroidism*, too much thyroxin is produced, causing the metabolic rate to speed up. This condition is marked by irritability, inability to sleep, bulging eyes, weight loss, and heat intolerance. The most common form of hyperthyroidism is Graves' disease, or toxic goiter. Enlargement of the thyroid gland is the most obvious sign of this disease. Hyperthyroidism has been implicated in the onset of osteoporosis in older persons. *Hypothyroidism* results from an insufficient production of thyroxin, and is marked by lethargy, extremely dry skin, cold intolerance, and weight gain. When this condition exists in a pregnant woman, her baby may be born with cretinism, a condition characterized by mental retardation and stunted growth.

While no genetic factor seems to play a role in these disorders, congenital and acquired factors do. Trauma, infection, exposure to radiation, and a diet poor in iodine are some of these. Iodine is needed by the thyroid gland for the production of thyroxin.

Managing Thyroid Disorders. Hyperthyroidism may be managed by either surgically removing part or all of the gland, or administering radioactive iodine or other drugs to inhibit the production of thyroxin. If it is necessary to totally remove the gland, the host will have to be treated with doses of thy-

Figure 3.9
Metabolism Diagram

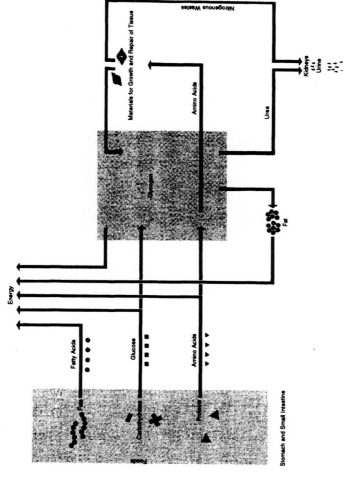

Source: Health For Better Living by M. Hurster. Englewood Cliffs, N.J.: Prentice-Hall, Inc., 1964, p. 138.

roxin for the rest of his or her life. Management of hypothyroidism also requires the lifelong administration of thyroxin.

Joint Disorders

Disorders involving the joints of the body, especially weight-bearing joints (hips, knees, and ankles), incapacitate well over 37 million people in the United States annually. While these disorders are not life-threatening, they have a considerable impact on the quality of life for those afflicted. At the very least, they may make it difficult and uncomfortable to perform simple tasks, such as dressing. A more serious scenario depicts them as making it impossible for a person to hold a steady job. Data from the *National Health Interview Survey* indicated that in 1985 the cost of these disorders, including medical care and lost wages, exceeded $21 billion. Clearly, this is a group of diseases deserving attention.

A *joint* is defined as a meeting, or articulation, of two bones. To permit the bones to articulate as intended, they are held in place by *connective tissue* in the form of ligaments. A membrane containing fluid encapsulates each joint to protect the surfaces of the articulating bones from friction produced as the joint is moved. This is the *synovial membrane*, and the fluid is *synovial fluid*.

Arthritis, or inflammation of a joint, is the generic term used to describe joint disorders. In general, an arthritic condition may arise either when the lubricating mechanism becomes inflamed (rheumatoid arthritis), or when the bones comprising the joint become eroded due to abuse (osteoarthritis).

Rheumatoid arthritis is characterized by redness, swelling, tenderness of the joint, stiffness, and pain on movement. This condition may affect any joint in the body. Two to three times as many females are affected as males, and the prevalence increases with age. This is an autoimmune disease, in which genetic factors seem to play an important role. It is also thought that ongoing exposure to minor bacterial infections may make the host more susceptible to this disease.

Osteoarthritis, also known as "wear and tear" arthritis, results from the gradual deterioration of the tissues designed to protect the joint. When the joint is exposed to repeated shock or impact, these tissues erode. This is the case in jogging, professional dance, and football, to name a few potentially joint-endangering activities. When erosion occurs, osteoarthritis sets in. This condition is accompanied by pain and tenderness. Precipitating factors include trauma to the joint, mechanical wear and tear, and a genetic predisposition.

There is no cure for either of these common forms of arthritis. Analgesics (pain killers) and muscle relaxants are usually prescribed. Weight loss, mild activity, and bracing of the afflicted part may also be prescribed.

Gout is another widely occurring joint disease. However, its etiology is quite different from arthritis. The body part involved in this condition is the big toe. Redness, swelling, and pain so extreme that the toe cannot bear to be covered, are the primary manifestations of gout. The cause, excessive production of and/or inability to excrete uric acid, is due to an inborn metabolic defect. Males are more subject to this condition. Other precipitating factors include hypertension, obesity, high alcohol consumption, and kidney disease. Management modalities include the use of anti-inflammatory drugs, drugs to increase excretion of uric acid, weight loss, and abstinence from alcohol.

Systemic lupus erythematosus (SLE) is an inflammatory, autoimmune disease that may affect many parts of the body, including the joints. SLE occurs more frequently in young women, and in Asians more than other races. Precipitating factors include a genetic predisposition and exposure to a variety of environmental factors, such as drugs, sunlight, and viruses. The condition is marked by fever, rash, loss of scalp hair, painful joints, pleurisy, skin lesions, and fatigue. Kidney involvement may also result.

Central Nervous System Disorders

The central nervous system consists of the brain, brain stem, and spinal cord. It is the repository of learning, memory, sensory responses, movement, coordination, and balance. In other words, it is the system that regulates most of, if not all, the attributes that enable us to function in the world. In addition, the brain stem, or medulla, regulates various responses that are *not* under voluntary control, such as breathing rate, heart rate, blood pressure, hunger, thirst, and emotions. These parts are illustrated in Figure 3.10.

Like any other part of the body, the central nervous system is subject to malfunctioning. The term *malfunctioning* may extend from a recognizable condition like multiple sclerosis or cerebral palsy, for which there are reasonable explanations, to a whole host of others which are not clear-cut, such as schizophrenia and depression. In this overview, we shall only touch on those central nervous system conditions for which we have some understanding of their prepathogenesis and pathogenesis stages.

Multiple sclerosis is a condition in which the covering of the nerve fibers leading to and from the brain deteriorates. As the nerve fibers are deprived of the protection afforded by this covering, scar tissue or lesions develop on them. This scarring results in only intermittent transmission of messages by the nerves, causing tremor and spasticity of the arms and legs. In addition, the host experiences weakness, stiffness, and incontinence, and will develop a staccato-like speech pattern. The cause of nerve covering deterioration is unknown, but a genetic predisposition is suspected. This is a terminal disease.

Cerebral Palsy is an inclusive term used to describe a group of conditions resulting from the development of lesions in the part of the central nervous system that regulates motor functions. As in multiple sclerosis, these lesions interfere with the smooth transmission of messages to the limbs, resulting in tremor, rigidity, and spasticity. The cause is unknown; how-

Figure 3.10
The Brain

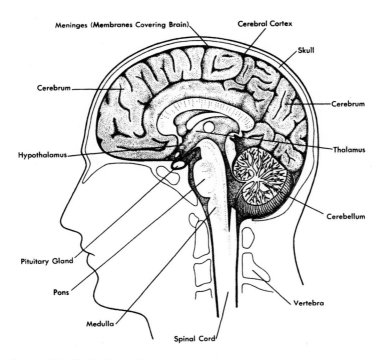

Meninges (Membranes Covering Brain)   Cerebral Cortex

Skull

Cerebrum

Cerebrum

Hypothalamus

Thalamus

Cerebellum

Pituitary Gland

Pons

Vertebra

Medulla

Spinal Cord

Source: *Health For Better Living* by M. Hurster. Englewood Cliffs, N.J.: Prentice-Hall, Inc., 1964, p. 194.

ever, it is thought that a complex interplay of inherited, congenital, and postnatal factors may be responsible for the onset
of this disease. Many of these factors can be attributed to inadequate prenatal care, prematurity, and complications arising
during the delivery process. Infants and young children are
most frequently affected, and males more often than females.
Lifelong speech, physical, and occupational therapy, along with
administration of drugs will be needed by the afflicted person.

Epilepsy is an incurable, intermittent brain disorder characterized by sudden, temporary episodes of seizures. Occurring

more frequently in males, its cause is undetermined. Two classes of seizure may occur: grand mal and petit mal. In both, consciousness is lost; however, in some cases of petit mal, it may be of such short duration as to go unnoticed. In grand mal, the loss of consciousness may be for an extended period of time, and accompanied by frothing at the mouth and spasms. Episodes are triggered by abnormal electrical discharges within the brain. Control of this disorder is achieved through drug therapy.

Factors implicated in the onset of epilepsy have been classified as strong, moderate, and suspected. *Strong precipitating factors* include: brain injury, central nervous system infections, structural brain abnormalities in the newborn, and anoxia (lack of sufficient oxygen) during the gestation period. *Moderate risk factors* include alcoholism and heroin usage by the mother during pregnancy. A genetic predisposition to epilepsy and development of multiple sclerosis in later life are also considered to be moderate risk factors. Aging is a suspected risk factor.

Alzheimer's is a disease in which aging is the primary risk factor. A genetic predisposition has also been identified as a risk factor. The highest incidence of Alzheimer's is among people in their ninth decade. In Stage I the following changes occur: mild memory loss, a decline in the ability to make spatial judgments, and slight personality changes. Stage II is identified by a worsening of Stage I changes, as well as restlessness and intermittent loss of the ability to speak. Stage III is marked by further deterioration of all mental, emotional, and physical functions, concluding in death. These changes are due to atrophy of brain tissue.

Parkinson's disease and amyotrophic lateral sclerosis (ALS) are two central nervous system diseases in which motor function is impaired. In Parkinson's disease, this impairment takes the form of tremors, stiffness, and slowness of movement. ALS is marked by weakness, twitching, and uncontrolled spasms, all of which worsen over time. The progression of Parkinson's disease can be controlled by medication. However, there is no way to halt the progression of ALS, which will end in death. The motor function impairment that occurs in both of these diseases is due to degeneration of nerves connecting the muscles with the brain, the cause of which is unknown.

Nutrition-Related Diseases

Although the diseases included under this heading are non-communicable, they differ in that most nutrition-related diseases can be cured. As the heading suggests, these diseases have to do with a person's level of nutrition. Daily ingestion of the recommended quantities of required nutrients is the key to preventing their onset.

Prevention. In order to prevent a nutritional disease, we need to know what our *recommended daily nutritional needs* are, and which foods will satisfy them. Nutrition information has been made readily available by both the public and private sectors. The U.S. Department of Agriculture and the U.S. Department of Health and Human Services have distributed a number of guides for healthy eating, including the Food Guide Pyramid (Figure 3.11). These publications have been augmented by numerous charts and informational pamphlets from the American Heart Association, the American Cancer Society, and the American Dietetic Association. The media have also contributed to the wealth of nutrition information available to the American public.

In spite of these efforts, Americans continue to ingest too much salt, sugar, and fat, and not enough fresh fruits and vegetables. Subsequently, it comes as no surprise that almost one-third of the U.S. population is overweight, and diseases with a nutritional base, such as heart disease, hypertension, some cancers, and diabetes, rank among our major health problems. Our early understanding of nutrition and its relationship to disease fostered the perception of nutrition-related diseases as being primarily "deficiency diseases." This led to them being identified as vitamin-, mineral-, and protein-deficiency diseases. As

Figure 3.11
Food Pyramid

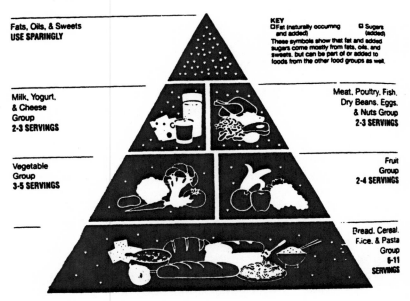

our knowledge grew, it became clear that nutrition serves other functions in the body besides preventing disease.

Functions of Food. These are: (1) providing a source of energy, (2) providing materials needed for growth and repair, and (3) providing materials needed to regulate body processes.

Providing a Source of Energy. All cells of the body require energy to function. The nutrients (*carbohydrates, proteins,* and *fats*) are the primary energy sources for the body. Through a complicated oxidation process known as the Krebs cycle, these nutrients are broken down into *glucose,* a simple sugar which serves as the body's fuel. This process yields energy in the form of calories. Heat is always released as a by-product of oxidation, and is measured in terms of calories. A calorie has been defined as the amount of heat needed to raise the temperature of one kilogram of water, one degree centigrade. Carbohydrates yield

4.1 calories per gram, proteins 4.1 calories per gram, and fats 9.1 calories per gram.

Inadequate Energy Intake. When the energy intake is inadequate, cellular activity will slow down. Initially, this will be manifested by lassitude, weakness, inattentiveness, irritability, and shortness of breath. These are signs associated with *hypoglycemia*, a condition in which there is a low blood level of glucose. Hypoglycemia is a common problem for people who fail to eat an adequate breakfast. For nondiabetics, hypoglycemia is a period of transitory discomfort—one which will disappear when they ingest some food. For diabetics, however, the appearance of these signs means that insulin intake has exceeded the level of glucose in the blood and could produce a condition of *insulin shock*. In insulin shock, all body functions are slowed down due to unavailability of energy. If the condition is not quickly reversed, death could ensue. Immediate ingestion of a source of quick energy, such as orange juice or a sugar cube, is essential to keep insulin shock from progressing.

A blood glucose reading of less than 70 mg marks the start of hypoglycemia. When it exceeds 140 mg, a condition of *hyperglycemia* is said to exist. This is one of the warning signs of diabetes. However, even after diabetes has been diagnosed and treatment prescribed, the diabetic needs to be alert for signs of hyperglycemia. These include drowsiness, blurred vision, nausea, rapid breathing, and a fruity odor of the breath, indicating an insufficient quantity of insulin to oxidize glucose. Failure to adminster insulin quickly will lead to *diabetic coma*, a life-threatening condition. Figure 3.12 illustrates how the body uses glucose in three different conditions.

Providing Materials for Growth and Repair. The processes of growth and repair are lifelong, and depend on an ongoing supply of protein, selected vitamins, and minerals. The required daily amounts of each nutrient vary with respect to age and activity level, but there is no period in the lifespan when growth and repair do not take place.

Figure 3.12
Glucose Usage

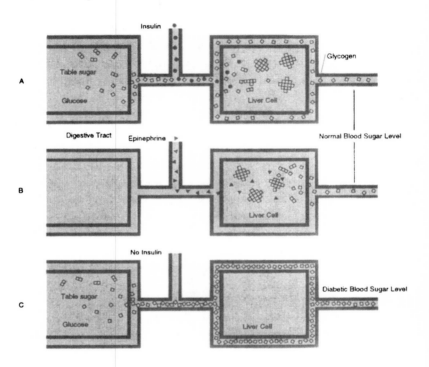

Source: Health For Better Living by M. Hurster. Englewood Cliffs, N.J.: Prentice-Hall, Inc., 1964, p. 284.

Protein is made of *amino acids*, which serve as the building blocks of each cell, and are essential for both growth and repair. Food sources of protein include meats, fish, eggs, legumes, milk, and grains. Protein deficiency may lead to stunted growth, mental retardation, and shortened life span. It is especially important that the pregnant woman has a diet rich in protein so she can satisfy both her baby's growth needs and her own.

Vitamins A, D, G, and *B-12* are also essential to normal growth and repair. Chart 3.4 indicates how they contribute, and in which foods they may be found.

Calcium and *phosphorous* are two minerals required for the normal development of bones and teeth. The need for them is greatest during the bone and teeth-forming years, as well as during pregnancy and the lactation period. Their role in preventing osteoporosis is unclear. For the body to absorb calcium and phosphorous, vitamin D must be present. Rickets is the deficiency disease that results when any of these is lacking. An infant deficient in these nutrients may be born with a deformed skeleton.

Providing Materials Needed to Regulate Body Processes. For the body to function correctly, it is essential that its internal environment be in a state of chemical balance, or *homeostasis*. Homeostasis is principally orchestrated by the nervous and endocrine systems working in concert with body organs and tissues. Together, they regulate the following homeostatic features: pH of the body, diffusion, osmosis, and temperature. They, in turn, need various nutrients to manufacture the compounds which impact homeostasis. Water, sodium, iodine, iron, and vitamins B-1, B-6, C, K, and niacin are the principal nutrients involved in maintaining homeostasis.

Water comprises two-thirds of the body, and is essential to the structure and function of every cell. It makes up the major part of the blood, urine, and all body secretions. Without it these body fluids would not exist, and the functions they perform would cease. Loss of 10 percent of body water is a serious threat to life; loss of 20 percent is fatal.

Sodium is the chief factor in maintenance of normal osmotic and diffusion pressures. It does this by causing the body to hold water in the spaces between the cells so that materials can pass into and out of them. While this represents a vital contribution to the body's functioning, sodium is something of a two-edged sword; ingestion of too much leads to over-retention of water by the cells, and subsequently to edema,

Vitamin Facts

Vitamin	U.S. RDA*	Best Sources	Functions	Deficiency Symptoms	Toxic?	Processing Tips	Did You Know?
A (carotene)	5000 IU/day	Yellow or orange fruits & vegetables, fortified oatmeal, green leafy vegetables, liver, dairy products	Formation & maintenance of skin, hair, & mucous membranes; helps us to see in dim light; bone & tooth growth	Night blindness, dry & scaly skin, frequent fatigue	Yes, in high doses, but beta-carotene is nontoxic.	Serve fruits & vegetables raw & keep covered & refrigerated. Steam veggies; broil, bake, or braise meats.	Lowfat & skim milks are often fortified with Vitamin A, which is removed with the fat.
B_1 (thiamine)	1.5 mg/day	Fortified cereals & oatmeals, meats, rice, & pasta, whole grains, liver	Helps body release energy from carbohydrates during metabolism; growth & muscle tone	Heart irregularity, fatigue, nerve disorders, mental confusion	No, high doses are excreted by the kidneys.	Don't rinse rice or pasta before & after cooking. Cook in minimal water.	Pasta & breads made of refined flours have B_1 added since it is lost in the milling process.
B_2 (riboflavin)	1.7 mg/day	Whole grains, green leafy vegetables, organ meats, milk & eggs	Helps body release energy from protein, fat, & carbohydrates during metabolism	Cracks in corners of mouth, skin rash, anemia	No toxic effects reported.	Store foods in containers that light cannot enter; cook vegetables in minimal water; roast or broil meats.	Most ready-to-eat cereals are fortified with 25% of the U.S. RDA for B_2.
B_6 (pyridoxine)	2 mg/day	Fish, poultry, lean meats, bananas, prunes, dried beans, whole grains, avocados	Helps build body tissue & aids in metabolism of protein	Convulsions, dermatitis, muscular weakness, skin cracks, anemia	Long-term megadoses may cause nerve damage in hands & feet.	Serve fruits raw or cook for shortest time in little water; roast or broil meats.	Since B_6 aids in use of protein in the body, the need for B_6 increases with protein intake.
B_{12} (cobalamin)	6 mcg/day	Meats, milk products, seafood	Aids cell development, functioning of the nervous system, & the metabolism of protein & fat	Anemia, nervousness, fatigue, &, in some cases, neuritis & brain degeneration	No toxic effects reported.	Roast or broil meat & fish.	Vegetarians who don't eat any animal products may need a supplement.
Biotin	0.3 mg/day	Cereal/grain products, yeast, legumes, liver	Involved in metabolism of protein, fats, & carbohydrates	Nausea, vomiting, depression, hair loss, dry, scaly skin	No toxic effects reported.	Storage, processing, & cooking do not appear to affect this vitamin.	Biotin deficiency is extremely rare in the U.S.
Folic Acid	0.4 mg/day	Green leafy vegetables, organ meats, dried peas, beans & lentils	Aids in genetic material development & involved in red blood cell production	Gastrointestinal disorders, anemia, cracks on lips	Some evidence of toxicity in large doses.	Store vegetables in refrigerator & steam, boil, or simmer in minimal water.	Deficiencies can occur in premature infants & pregnant women.

Vitamin	RDA	Sources	Functions	Deficiency Symptoms	Toxicity	Storage/Preparation	Notes
Niacin	20 mg/day	Meat, poultry, fish, enriched cereals, peanuts, potatoes, dairy products, eggs	Involved in carbohydrate, protein, & fat metabolism	Skin disorders, diarrhea, indigestion, general fatigue	Nicotinic acid form should be taken only under doctor's care.	Roast or broil beef, veal, lamb, & poultry. Cook potatoes in minimal water.	Niacin is formed in the body by converting an amino acid found in proteins.
Pantothenic Acid	10/mg/day	Lean meats, whole grains, legumes, vegetables, fruits	Helps in the release of energy from fats & carbohydrates	Fatigue, vomiting, stomach stress, infections, muscle cramps	No toxic effects reported.	Eat fruits & vegetables raw.	It is believed some pantothenic acid is produced in the G.I. tract.
C (ascorbic acid)	60 mg/day	Citrus fruits, berries, & vegetables—especially peppers	Essential for structure of bones, cartilage, muscle & blood vessels. Also helps maintain capillaries & gums & aids in absorption of iron	Swollen or bleeding gums, slow wound healing, fatigue/ depression, poor digestion	Intakes of one gram or more can cause nausea, cramps, & diarrhea.	Do not store or soak fruits & vegetables in water. Refrigerate juices & store only 2–3 days.	Smokers may benefit from an increased intake of Vitamin C.
D	400 IU/day	Fortified milk, sunlight, fish, eggs, butter, fortified margarine	Aids in bone & tooth formation; helps maintain heart action & nervous system	In children: rickets & other bone deformities. In adults: calcium loss from bones	High intakes may cause diarrhea & weight loss.	Storage, processing, & cooking do not appear to affect this vitamin.	Sunlight starts Vitamin D production in the skin.
E	30 IU/day	Fortified & multi-grain cereals, peanuts, wheat germ, vegetable oils, green leafy vegetables	Protects blood cells, body tissue, & essential fatty acids from harmful destruction in the body	Muscular wasting, nerve damage, anemia, reproductive failure	Relatively nontoxic.	Store in airtight containers away from light.	Most fortified cereals have 40% of the RDA.
K	**	Green leafy vegetables, fruit, dairy & grain products	Essential for blood clotting functions	Bleeding disorders in newborn infants & those on blood-thinning medications	Not toxic as found in food.	Store in containers away from light.	Vitamin K is also formed by bacteria in the colon.

Source: This chart may be reprinted without permission. Poster-size versions of the chart are available upon request. Please write to Nestlé Information Services. Information for this chart was obtained from the Food and Drug Administration, the American Institute for Cancer Research and the United States Department of Agriculture/Human Nutrition Information Service.

* For adults and children over four. IU=international units, mg=milligrams, mcg=micrograms
** There is no U.S. RDA for Vitamin K, however the recommended dietary allowance is 1 mcg/kg of body weight.

weight gain, and elevated blood pressure. Sodium is present in every food; hence, the term, *salt free* is a misnomer.

Iodine's role in the production of thyroxin has already been discussed. Without ample quantities of iodine, the thyroid gland is incapable of producing thyroxin, the hormone responsible for regulating the body's metabolic rate. An abnormal metabolic rate will upset the homeostasis of the entire body. Iodine occurs naturally in all saltwater fish, and in fruits and vegetables grown in coastal regions. It has been added to table salt for the benefit of those who lack access to natural food sources of iodine.

Iron is required by the red blood cells for the production of hemoglobin. Without hemoglobin, the red blood cells would be unable to carry oxygen; thus, body cells would be incapable of oxidizing glucose, and therefore lack the fuel needed to continue functioning. A person with this condition, *iron deficiency anemia*, tires easily, gets out of breath at the slightest exertion, and often feels light-headed. By adding iron-rich foods to the diet, such as liver, eggs, and green leafy vegetables, this condition can be alleviated. There are several other forms of anemia not related to iron deficiency, such as might arise temporarily during menstruation, or due to blood loss following an accident. In *pernicious anemia*, an insufficient number of red blood cells is produced, and those that are produced fail to mature and are incapable of carrying oxygen. Another form of anemia results from destruction of bone marrow due to radiation.

Vitamin B-1, or *thiamine*, is needed for the proper utilization of carbohydrates. Thiamine deficiency weakens all muscle tissue, and may lead to heart failure. Other less life-threatening consequences of this deficiency include: polyneuritis (inflammation of the nerve coverings), indigestion, constipation, nausea, and loss of appetite. Good food sources for thiamine are pork, whole grains, nuts, and legumes.

Niacin also plays an important role in delivery of oxygen to the cells. It frees oxygen from the hemoglobin, thus facilitating its diffusion into the cells, which is essential to cell function. Niacin may be found in meats, milk, green leafy vegetables, and legumes.

Vitamin B-6, or *pyridoxine,* is needed for protein metabolism and antibody production. Cells cannot survive without protein, and antibodies are essential in our ability to combat communicable diseases. Pyridoxine is found in meat, fish, liver, and wheat germ.

Vitamin C, or *ascorbic acid,* is best known as a scurvy preventive. However, it performs several other functions of equal importance. One of these is to act as a cell-cementing substance which enhances the integrity of the cell wall. Another is to maintain a normal concentration of iron in the blood. Bruising easily, and gums that readily bleed may be signs of vitamin C deficiency. Citrus fruits, tomatoes, and green leafy vegetables are good sources of this vitamin, which is highly fragile; exposure to air and heat will cause loss of vitamin C from the foods containing it.

Vitamin K plays a vital role in blood clotting. It is needed by the liver for the formation of prothrombin and its conversion into thrombin, a principal clotting element of the blood.

Allergies

Allergies are diseases of *hypersensitivity* and usually occur in response to an exogenous factor, such as pollen, animal dander, drugs, certain foods, and dust. There are four types of hypersensitivity reactions: (1) immediate or anaphylactic, (2) cytotoxic, (3) complex-mediated, and (4) cell-mediated or delayed.

Immediate or *anaphylactic hypersensitivity* is marked by an oversecretion of mucus and a release of histamine. The histamine causes the bronchi in the lungs to constrict, making breathing difficult, and the oversecretion of mucus further exacerbates the problem by clogging the breathing passages. A person suffering from this reaction may also develop hives during the episode. Asthma, hay fever, eczema, and urticaria are conditions arising from this type of hypersensitivity, and fatal systemic anaphylaxis is an extreme response to it.

Cytotoxic hypersensitivity is a condition in which antibodies attack their antigens, as well as normal cells and tissue. This is the type of allergic reaction that creates problems in blood transfusions and organ transplants. It also occurs in Rh factor incompatibility between mother and fetus. In this condition, the mother lacks the Rh factor, a genetically determined blood component, while the fetus she is carrying has the Rh factor. People who have the factor are designated as being Rh-positive; those lacking it as Rh-negative. During pregnancy, the Rh factor may pass through the placenta from fetus to mother, but since the factor is recognized by the mother's immune system as a foreign element, her body produces antibodies in response to it. These antibodies then travel back to the fetus via the placenta, and proceed to destroy its red blood cells. If this transfer occurs early in pregnancy, the fetus may die; if it takes place late in pregnancy, the baby will be born with edema, a condition in which the tissues are swollen with accumulated fluids. A baby born with edema will probably be mentally re-tarded since it will have impacted brain tissue. If the transfer occurs just before delivery, the baby will be born jaundiced. Of these three Rh factor incompatibility consequences, only the last one can be ameliorated. By transfusing out the baby's Rh-positive blood, and transfusing in Rh-negative, the jaundice will be relieved, and in time, the baby will regenerate the Rh factor since he or she has its gene.

Complex-mediated hypersensitivity is a reaction in which an-tibodies combine with antigens and complement to form com-plexes which get trapped in the small blood vessels of the kidneys, joints, lungs, and skin. These complexes interfere with the ability of these body parts to function normally, by creating an acute inflammatory response in them. SLE, rheumatoid ar-thritis, rheumatic fever, and rheumatic heart are examples of conditions arising from this type of reaction.

Cell-mediated or *delayed hypersensitivity* results when antibodies that are not fully developed and have been stored within body cells become activated after lengthy exposure to an antigen. Contact dermatitis, drug sensitivity, and certain infection allergies are examples of this type of reaction. They may appear without any warning and often are not immediately recognized as delayed hypersensitivity reactions.

Psychogenic or Functional Disorders

This group of disorders is closely associated with psychic stress resulting from social, psychological, and environmental factors. They not only interfere with a person's life-style, but also substantially contribute to other diseases and often determine the course of a disease. Psychogenic disorders reflect the power of the mind to affect the health of the body. They involve the process of *somatization*, whereby an emotional or mental state changes a physiological function. Peptic ulcer, ulcerative colitis, spastic colon, asthma, and dermatitis are examples of psychogenic disorders.

Brief Description of Some Conditions of Special Concern to Children

Hemophilia is an inherited coagulation disorder in which the blood fails to clot. It is passed from the mother to her male offspring. The hemophiliac bruises easily, is subject to frequent nosebleeds, and represents a serious surgical risk.

Down's syndrome is due to a chromosomal defect. Children born with this condition are mentally retarded, have a mongoloid facial appearance, and a shortened life span.

Muscular dystrophy is a group of diseases characterized by progressive muscle wasting and weakness. A chromosomal defect is responsible for this disease.

Sickle-cell disease is characterized by sickle-shaped red blood cells. This shape makes it difficult for them to pass through the capillaries. They congregate there, obstructing the flow of blood and interfering with the capillaries' transfer function. This leads to severe pain, ulceration of the skin, shortness of breath, and myocardial infarction. African Americans are especially prone to this disease.

Phenylketonuria, or *PKU*, is a disorder in which the body lacks the enzyme *phenylalanine*, which is needed for the metabolism of protein. The disease appears at birth, and can be treated by administration of the missing enzyme. Failure to do this will lead to abnormal brain development and mental retardation.

Spina bifida is a congenital defect in which the bones of the skull and vertebral column fail to fuse, leading to major problems of motor and speech development, as well as the ability to learn.

Cleft palate/cleft lip is due to genetic factors which cause malformation of the palate and lip. The defect may be unilateral or bilateral.

Fetal alcohol syndrome (FAS) is the result of maternal alcoholism. Effects on the fetus include: severe mental retardation, heart defects, and immunodeficiency. FAS is the third leading cause of mental retardation in newborns.

Mental retardation is a learning deficit which can result from prenatal infection, birth trauma, FAS, and a variety of inherited factors. In general, a person is considered mentally retarded if his or her IQ is less than 100.

Lead poisoning, or *plumbism*, is a condition to which children are especially susceptible because of their small body size. Lead, a heavy metal, can enter the body via ingestion, inhalation, or absorption. Once in the body, it damages membranes, causes the brain to swell, and injures nerves and bones. Anemia, mental retardation, and muscle weakness are some of the results of untreated lead poisoning. Anemia and muscle weakness can be reversed with proper treatment.

SUMMARY

Non-communicable diseases account for the three leading causes of death in the United States. Unlike communicable diseases, for which specific causes can be identified, non-communicable diseases have no single causative factor. Instead, they are the products of a variety of precipitating or risk factors, which range from heredity to aging, life-style, stress, and exposure to environmental hazards. Some of these factors cannot be changed, and therefore remain risks. Others, however, are subject to modification and even elimination. Their continued high incidence and prevalence rates are a reflection of our lack of will to both alter our personal life-styles, and allocate the necessary resources to bring these diseases under control. The prepathogenesis of non-communicable diseases involves the interaction of the host with risk factors which, with few exceptions, will progress to the pathogenesis stage. Since most non-communicable diseases are incurable, preventing them is of the utmost importance.

LEARNING OBJECTIVES

From this discussion of non-communicable diseases, the student will be able to:

1. define the term *non-communicable disease.*
2. give an example of a non-communicable disease for each grouping covered in the text.
3. explain the term *precipitating* or *risk factor* with respect to non-communicable disease.
4. list five groups of risk factors relating to non-communicable disease.
5. identify those risk factors over which the host has control, and describe the nature of that control.

6. identify the parts of the circulatory system, and explain their roles in the body.

7. identify the parts of the respiratory system, and explain their roles in the body.

8. identify the parts of the central nervous system, and explain their roles in the body.

9. differentiate between the terms *inherited, congenital*, and *acquired*, as related to risk factors, and give an example of each.

10. define the term *prematurity*, and identify three ways in which it may affect the baby.

REFERENCES

Becker, M., ed. *The Health Belief Model and Personal Health Behavior*. Thoroughfare, NJ: Slack, 1974.

Brownson, R. C., P. L. Remington, and J. R. Davis, eds. *Chronic Disease Epidemiology and Control*. Washington, DC: American Public Health Association, 1993.

Ciesielski, P. F. *Major Chronic Diseases*. Guilford, CT: The Dushkin Publishing Group, 1992.

Dickey, L. L., H. M. Griffith, and D. B. Kamerow. "Put Prevention Into Practice." In *Clinician's Handbook of Preventive Services*. DHHS/PHS, Office of Disease Prevention and Health Promotion, 1994.

Edlin, G., E. Golanty, and K. McCormack Brown. *Health and Wellness*. 5th ed. Boston: Jones and Bartlett Publishers, 1996.

Fardy, P. S., J. Magel, and M. Hurster, et al. "Prevalence of Coronary Artery Disease Risk Factors in Minority Adolescents: A Feasibility Study." *J. Cardiopulmonary Rehab.* 9: 404, 1989.

Fardy, P. S., R. E. C. White, L. T. Clark, and M. Hurster, et al. "Coronary Risk Factors and Health Behaviors in a Diverse Ethnic and Cultural Population of Adolescents: A Gender Comparison." *J. Cardiopulmonary Rehab.* 14: 52–60, 1994.

———. "Health Promotion in Minority Adolescents." *J. Cardiopulmonary Rehab.* 15: 65–72, 1995.

Guyton, A. C., and J. E. Hall. *Textbook of Medical Physiology*. 9th ed. Philadelphia: W. B. Saunders, 1995.

Kandel, D., P. Wu, and M. Davies. "Maternal Smoking During Pregnancy and Smoking by Adolescent Daughters." *AJPH* 84: 1407–13, 1994.

Kerson, T. S., and L. A. Kerson. *Understanding Chronic Illness*. New York: The Free Press, 1985.

Koop, C. E. "Editorial: A Personal Role in Health Care Reform." *AJPH* 85: 759, 1995.

Kotelchuck, M. "The Adequacy of Prenatal Care Utilization Index: Its U.S. Distribution and Association with Low Birthweight." *AJPH* 84: 1486–88, 1994.

Krebs-Smith, S. M., A. Cook, and A. Subar, et al. "U.S. Adults' Fruit and Vegetable Intakes, 1989 to 1991: A Revised Baseline for the Healthy People 2000 Objective." *AJPH* 85: 1612–28, 1995.

Land, G. H., and J. W. Stockbauer. "Smoking and Pregnancy Outcome: Trends among Black Teenage Mothers in Missouri." *AJPH* 83: 1121–24, 1993.

Marshall, J. "Editorial: Improving Americans' Diet—Setting Public Policy with Limited Knowledge." *AJPH* 85: 1609–10, 1995.

Public Health Service. "Healthy People 2000. National Health Promotion and Disease Prevention Objectives." Washington, DC: U.S. Dept. of Health and Human Services, 1991. DHHS Publication PHS 91: 50212.

Purtilo, D. T., and R. B. Purtilo. *A Survey of Human Diseases.* Boston: Little, Brown Co., 1989.

Shea, S. "Editorial: Hypertension Control." *AJPH* 84: 1725–26, 1994.

Sheldon, H. *Boyd's Introduction to the Study of Disease.* Philadelphia: Lea and Febiger, 1984.

Waisbren, S. E., and B. D. Hamilton, et al. "Psychosocial Factors in Maternal Phenylketonuria: Women's Adherence to Medical Recommendations." *AJPH* 85: 1636–40, 1995.

4

ROLES OF THE INDIVIDUAL, THE COMMUNITY, AND THE GOVERNMENT IN DISEASE PREVENTION

The former surgeon general of the United States, C. Everett Koop, has said that "diseases are of two types: those we develop inadvertently and those we bring upon ourselves by failure to practice preventive measures. Preventable illness makes up approximately 70% of the burden of illness and associated costs." Clearly, it behooves us to do all we can to prevent disease. This task represents a shared responsibility on the parts of the individual, the community, and the government. However, this is by no means an equal sharing. There is only so much the individual acting alone can do to protect him or herself from pathogens and environmental hazards. Likewise, there is just so much that a single community can do to protect its citizens. And while the government can enact disease-prevention legislation and try to enforce it, the effectiveness of these efforts requires the cooperation/compliance of individuals and communities. How an individual and/or community will respond depends largely on how well informed each is about the nature of the disease hazard, and whether the steps or actions needed to prevent the hazard are perceived to be more beneficial than the cost or effort involved in taking them.

Unfortunately, being well informed about *how* to prevent a disease does not always result in behavior that *will* prevent it. It follows, therefore, that while education about disease prevention is an important first step, it should not be regarded as the sole method of addressing this goal. Individuals do not always act in their own best health interests, even when they know better. And when it comes to the health interests of the public at large, individuals may be even less inclined to do so.

EDUCATION: THE FIRST STEP

We are not born with a knowledge of how to prevent disease; these steps must be learned, and their importance explained. Primary disease prevention measures may be subsumed under the heading of good hygiene, and include: washing hands before eating and after using the toilet, keeping the body clean, getting enough rest, having a well-balanced diet, getting adequate exercise, dressing appropriately for the weather, avoiding sources of contagion as much as possible, coping with stress effectively, not smoking, not using drugs, getting regular medical and dental checkups, and complying with physicians' and dentists' advice. Old-fashioned as these practices may seem, they are nevertheless highly effective ways for the individual to keep from falling ill. They are also cost-effective in that preventing the onset of a disease is far less expensive and time-consuming in the long run than attempting to cure it.

The most propitious time to acquire good hygiene practices is childhood. It follows, therefore, that these practices should comprise a substantial part of the elementary school health education program, which should be one of the major components of the elementary school curriculum. And, because of its importance to the future well-being of the child, the program should be under the direction of a health education specialist.

ROLE OF PARENTS AND THE SCHOOL AS CHANGE AGENTS

Since a child spends his or her most impressionable years under the supervision of parents and teachers, the responsibility for inculcating good preventive habits rests predominantly with them. Good hygiene practices can become lifelong habits if learned early in life. Habits acquired in childhood become deeply imbedded in a person's life-style, are the least amenable to change later in life, and are likely to remain with the person for the rest of his or her life. For parents and teachers to succeed in teaching good hygiene practices, they must share the same health-related goals, and encourage the same health practices so the child does not receive conflicting messages. Being good role models themselves; that is, doing what they are telling the child to do, is one way of encouraging good hygiene practices. Reinforcing the desired behavior by avoiding disparity between what is taught in school and what is practiced at home is another way of getting the message across. Rules of good health behavior should be established, and compliance encouraged.

The School Health Council

Parents and teachers can effectively work together toward these goals if guidelines are provided. A school health council comprised of representatives from the teaching staff, parents' association, school administration, and student body represents one way of doing this. The presence of such a group in the school setting affords ongoing opportunity for monitoring the health status of the school community, identifying school health problems that need to be addressed, and taking appropriate action with respect to these problems. Ideally, the school health council should be headed by a *professional health educator* because he or she will have a broad-based understanding of health problems, and the knowledge and expertise needed to solve them. *Administrative support and input* are crucial to the effectiveness of the council, because necessities such as funding and the willingness to include health-related programs and activities in the school schedule and curriculum must be obtained from the school administration. *Parental participation* on the council is also critical to its success because there must be carry-over from the school to the home if the health teachings and sound health habits are to be firmly inculcated. For this to occur, parents need to play an active role in the decision-making processes of the council, thereby acquiring a sense of ownership in the school health program and a deeper level of commitment to the goals of the council. *Student participation* is necessary for these same reasons. And it is entirely appropriate that there be student input on the council, since the school health program is designed for the students.

The School Administration

In addition to supporting the school health council, the administration also has responsibility for complying with all governmental regulations regarding the health and safety of pupils and teachers. With respect to primary prevention, these include: making sure all pupils have been immunized against such childhood diseases as diphtheria, polio, tetanus, pertussis, measles, mumps, and rubella before being admitted to school; making sure the physical environment of the school is free from environmental hazards which may contribute to disease or injury; and working cooperatively with other community organizations and resources with respect to disease prevention.

For these models of cooperation and collaboration to work, parents, teachers, and school administrators must also be knowledgeable about disease prevention. This raises the question of how to educate them so they can be effective teachers and role models for the children in their care. Elementary school teachers could and should be required to take at least one course in disease prevention as part of their undergraduate preparation. School administrators should also be required to take such a course prior to being licensed. Unfortunately, the education of parents cannot be mandated and specified in this way. This task, therefore, falls to a variety of community resources, such as schools, the public health department, voluntary health agencies, providers of health care, and the media. While these resources are capable, they tend to function unilaterally, focusing only on the disease entity they represent, and reaching only those already prevention-minded and somewhat knowledgeable about disease. Those who may be most at risk from disease because of lack of access to health care are often the very ones not reached by disease prevention information sources.

ROLE OF OTHER COMMUNITY RESOURCES AS CHANGE AGENTS

Most communities have access to a variety of health information sources, some in the private sector and some in the public sector.

Private Sector Resources

Among those in the private sector whose primary function is the dispensing of health information are *voluntary health agencies*. These not-for-profit organizations are committed to providing the public with accurate, current information about the disease entity on which they focus. Each has a research component which provides updated information on various aspects of the disease, as well as an outreach program through which information is transmitted to the public. Outreach is achieved via printed materials, videotapes, and films, which are available to the public either at no cost or for a small fee. These materials are augmented by a cadre of knowledgeable speakers who are available to make presentations to schools and other community organizations free of charge, and who are trained to work with these groups in the planning and implementing of health-related programs for their constituents. Financial support for these agencies is solicited from the public via annual appeals, and grant-giving foundations, both private and governmental. Examples of voluntary health agencies include: the American Cancer Society, the American Lung Association, the American Heart Association, the March of Dimes, and the American Red Cross.

Local *provider organizations* such as hospitals, clinics, and HMOs also dispense information about disease prevention, even though their primary purpose is provision of care. They, too, distribute printed materials about various disease entities and offer lectures and seminars on health matters to area residents.

Insurance companies serve as another source of health information. The Prudential Insurance Company has a long history of educating the public about disease prevention through its many pamphlets and posters. More recently, Blue Cross/Blue Shield has incorporated health education into its organizational structure. Additionally, the Health Insurance Plan of greater New York has offered health education for its members since its inception.

Public Sector Resources

In addition to community schools, another important public sector health education resource is the *local public health department*, which supported by tax dollars, performs a multifaceted role in disease prevention. In addition to dispensing health information, it also monitors the community's health status; alerts it to potential health problems; provides a wide spectrum of preventive services, including immunizations and screening tests, either at no cost or for a nominal fee; oversees the sanitary conditions of public eating places, food handling, and preparation; is responsible for seeing that all standards included in the community's health code are being met; and maintains community records on mortality and morbidity rates.

While these services are the direct responsibility of the local public health department, they may be augmented by state and federal government aid and regulation. Both of these political entities exercise a considerable measure of control over the health of a given community by virtue of their funding capabilities, and ability to enact and enforce health-related legislation.

ROLE OF THE MEDIA AS CHANGE AGENT

Newspapers, magazines, radio, television, and now the internet, all transmit health information to the public. These resources represent a potentially excellent way to inform large numbers of people about the genesis of health problems, their dangers, how to keep from becoming their victim, and what to do should that condition arise. When the media report accurate, up-to-date information in an objective, nonsensational manner, they serve as a valuable community resource.

COMPLIANCE: THE NEXT STEP

Giving people information about disease prevention is, in one respect, the easy part of the mission to encourage positive health behavior. Getting them to actually change their behavior requires the change agent/planner to have an accurate picture of the target population and its available resources, as well as an understanding of the factors that underlie its behavior. Regardless of whether the change agent/planner is a parent, the school, community, or government, the following steps need to be taken. While the methods may vary depending on who the change agent/planner is, the goal remains the same— to change health behavior in a positive direction.

Learning About the Target Population

Clearly, it is incumbent on the change agent/planner to become as knowledgeable about the target population as possible. To accomplish this, a *needs assessment* should be conducted before any attempt to change behavior is made.

Needs Assessment. A needs assessment may be defined as a systematic procedure for identifying: (1) the characteristics and needs of an individual or community, (2) the resources available both within and outside of the community for meeting those needs, and (3) the barriers to satisfying them. The needs assessment provides the change agent/planner with an objective picture of what *needs* to be done and what *can* be done. This sort of analysis enables the planner to set priorities, maximize his or her resources, and select appropriate behavior change strategy.

The needs assessment is made up of three steps: (1) identifying the current health status of the target, (2) analyzing the health status information, and (3) prioritizing the steps needed to address the health problem.

Identification of the target's current health status may be accomplished in several ways. A review of official health records will objectively indicate the most pressing health needs. This information may, and probably should, be augmented by opinions elicited from the target population itself by means of surveys, questionnaires, community meetings, and focus groups. Although these sources may be subjective in nature, they are important for several reasons. First, they provide an emotional/personal dimension to health status, which official data are not designed to give. Second, they engage the target population in the change transaction at its earliest stage, arousing a feeling of ownership in the plan, which will encourage their participation and cooperation in its implementation.

In addition to taking the aforementioned steps, the change agent/planner should make his or her own on-site observation of the target population. Among the considerations that should be included are: what programs are already in place to address the identified health problems; and which are effective and which are not, along with the reasons for their success or failure.

Once this information has been collected, the change agent/planner needs to analyze it to identify any gaps that may exist in addressing the health problem. This analysis will provide a more realistic picture of the problem, and enable the change agent/planner to prioritize his or her efforts. Having done this, the next step will be to select those behavior-change strategies appropriate to the problem and the target population. A behavior-change strategy may be defined as a plan for bringing about change in the way something or someone is responded to. The plan is usually the tool of the change agent/planner, and the target of the plan is usually the individual or community whose behavior the planner seeks to change. An effective strategy will be based on an understanding of the factors that underlie behavior.

Bases of Behavior

Instinct. Behavior may be defined as an *instinctual response* to someone or something. At its most basic level, behavior is geared to the instinct for survival, to satisfy those needs which will make it possible for the individual/community to continue functioning. Food, shelter, and safety are examples of such needs. In Maslow's Hierarchy of Needs theory, he identifies five levels of human need, and states that need levels must be satisfied sequentially, beginning with the most basic. Unless this occurs, it will be impossible to bring about behavior change involving higher need levels. According to Maslow, the five need levels are: (1) food and shelter, (2) safety, (3) love, (4) self-esteem, and (5) self-actualization. It would be foolhardy to attempt to get a target population which is living from hand-to-mouth, barely satisfying the most basic need (level 1), to embark on an exercise regime designed to raise its level of physical fitness, a goal related most closely to self-actualization (level 5). In this case, the change agent/planner would be well advised to focus his or her efforts on another population, one whose lower-level needs are being met.

Another instinct that is associated with survival and serves as a determinant of behavior is the *fight or flight response.* When faced with a threat, some people will do everything in their power to avoid it. This flight response ranges from *denying* that a threat or problem exists, to simply throwing up one's hands in despair and declaring that nothing can be done about it. Others respond to threats/problems by first acknowledging their existence, and then attempting to deal with them; that is, by employing a fight response. When the flight response is resorted to, the pain or fear associated with the threat/problem may be temporarily allayed; but, in time, these feelings will return because the source has not been dealt with. In contrast, by employing a fight response, or taking action against the threat/problem, it may be removed or solved.

The consequences of either type of response with respect to a health concern are clear. By denying the existence of a health problem, and thereby taking no steps to alleviate or control it, the chances are very good that it will only worsen. Hence, a flight response in such a case is nonproductive. Conversely, by following a recommended course of action designed to alleviate or control the problem, it may be removed or, at least, modified.

In his Locus of Control theory, Rotter postulates that people tend to be either *internally* or *externally* controlled. An *internally controlled* person is one who views him or herself as being in charge of a situation, and his or her actions as being responsible for the outcome of a situation. Such a person tends to be independent and aggressive, a leader. In contrast, the *externally controlled* person views him or herself as the victim of circumstances, someone to whom things happen. The notion of being in control is completely foreign to such people. They tend to be dependent and acquiescent, followers. Of the two types, the externally controlled person might seem more amenable to changing his or her health behavior. However, while such a person may tend to be more receptive to a health message, the determination to act on it may be lacking, for externally controlled people usually rely on others to bring about change.

The internally controlled person, on the other hand, may offer more initial resistance to a proposed change. But once convinced of its value, he or she will take the necessary steps to effecting it. The change agent/planner needs to assess the overall nature of his or her target population to select the behavior-change strategies that will be most consonant with the target's locus of control.

Learning or Conditioning. Behavior may also be viewed as a *learned or conditioned response* that is shaped by parents, peers, and society throughout our lifetime, even during the gestation period. Edward Hall identifies three sources of influence that determine how we respond. The *earliest* of these sources originates from *parents*, and lays the foundation for how the child will perceive him or herself, his or her surroundings and the world in general, as well as how he or she will behave with respect to these entities. Prejudices, religious beliefs, cultural practices, ethical and moral standards, ethnic/racial identity, language, sex roles, manners, and basic hygiene practices are some of the learnings that parents pass on to their children and shape their behavior. Hall postulates that these learnings are transmitted throughout the child's formative years. What is learned at this time becomes deeply ingrained in the child's life-style, and is the most resistant to change. This is not to say that it can never be changed, but the time and effort needed to bring about change at this stage might be better directed at behaviors acquired later in life that are more amenable to change.

Hall goes on to say that the next source of influence comes from *association with peers*. He calls this the *imitative* stage, in which the child strives to gain acceptance from his or her peers by adopting their perceptions, behaviors, and beliefs. As the child begins to associate with other children in play situations, and especially upon entrance to school, he or she is introduced to different ways of believing, behaving, and thinking. The value system that had been instilled by the child's parents may be seriously challenged by these new influences, causing considerable turmoil in the child. This may manifest itself in rebellious behavior and disrupt the life of the family. Adolescence is the time in the child's life when rebellious behavior is most likely to occur. Hall maintains that the behaviors and values acquired during this period are not as deeply ingrained in the life-style as those acquired earlier in life, and therefore are more easily changed. Hall's third stage of conditioning refers to those skills and learnings acquired via *formal schooling*.

These are the least deeply ingrained in the life-style, and the most amenable to change.

If we accept Hall's theory, it follows that behavior-change efforts should be *initially* focused on behaviors learned during the formal schooling stage for the following reasons: (1) the efforts are more likely to succeed, (2) success of any magnitude fosters confidence in both the change agent/planner and the target population, and (3) success tends to encourage a spirit of teamwork between the two players involved in the change transaction. Once a measure of success has been achieved, and feelings of trust and togetherness have been engendered, the change agent/planner and the target population will be more inclined to work together and take on more challenging projects, such as those involving behaviors acquired during the imitative stage, and even those learned initially from parents.

Festinger's theory of Cognitive Dissonance represents another explanation of how learning/conditioning may shape behavior. Festinger says that for behavior change to take place, a state of dissonance must be created in the target population. Dissonance results when the target receives new information that is in conflict with, or disagrees with, information he or she already holds. This arouses uncertainty, unease, even guilt; these are feelings that cannot be tolerated indefinitely—they demand resolution by the target. At this moment, the target becomes ready to take action, and it is therefore the most propitious time for the change agent to intervene with a behavior-change strategy. This strategy should include both a plan for arousing dissonance and resolving it in a way that is consonant with positive health behavior.

Kurt Lewin views behavior as the sum of driving and restraining forces, which together create the sense of dissonance. He suggests that one way conflict/dissonance may be resolved is to: (1) strengthen the driving forces by emphasizing the reasons/factors mitigating for the desired health behavior, (2) reduce the restraining factors mitigating against the desired health behavior by allowing the target to release his or her feelings by talking them out, and (3) combine steps 1 and 2. He offers the Five-Phase Unfreeze-Refreeze theory as a way of bringing about positive health behavior. In Phase 1, the Unfreezing Phase, dissonance is aroused, thus making the target open to change. Phase 2 is the Problem-Diagnosis Phase; here the forces mitigating for and against change are evaluated, and possible intervention points identified. Phase 3 is the Goal-Setting Phase, in which a plausible plan of action is selected, and Phase 4, the New-Behavior Phase, involves implementation of the plan of action. Phase 5 is the Refreezing Phase, in which the new behavior becomes internalized.

Underlying Motivations. Behavior may also be viewed as a response to *underlying motivations.* The Health Belief Model, designed by Lewin, Rosenstock, and Festinger et al., identifies some of the motivations underlying health behavior. Health Belief Model, Version I, is an embodiment of several of Maslow's and Hall's beliefs, in that it demonstrates how need level and conditioning can interact to produce a given behavior. In Chart 4.1, Health Belief Model I, the interplay between individual perceptions and modifying factors, and the possible results of this interplay are shown. Individual perceptions refers to *how* the individual/community views a disease threat, and modifying factors refers to *factors that contribute* to the way the disease threat is perceived. Hence, the individual/community may or may not regard the disease threat as something they need to be concerned about; this is their perception of the threat. In the process of assessing it, they may have asked the following questions: What are the chances that I/we will acquire this disease? If the chances are slight, is it worth the effort, time, and money to take the steps needed to prevent the disease? How serious is the disease? If it isn't serious, is it necessary to take the preventive steps that are recommended?

In answering these questions, the individual and the community are weighing the importance of taking preventive action from the perspective of the need level on which they are currently functioning, and from the way they have been con-

Chart 4.1
Health Belief Model I

INDIVIDUAL PERCEPTIONS	MODIFYING FACTORS	LIKELIHOOD OF ACTION
	Demographic variables: age, sex, ethnicity, etc.	Perceived benefits of action
Perceived Susceptibility of Disease "x"	Sociopsychological variables: personality, social class, peer and reference group pressures, etc.	MINUS
Perceived Seriousness of Disease "x"	Perceived Threat of Disease "x"	Perceived barriers to action
	<u>Cues to Action</u> Mass Media Campaigns Advise from others Reminder card from physician/dentist Illness of friend or family member	Likelihood of taking recommended action

Source: The Health Belief Model and Personal Health Behavior by M. Becker, ed. Thoroughfare, N.J.: Slack, 1974.

ditioned to view disease. If the need level on which they are functioning is a low one, such as food, shelter, or safety, and if they have been conditioned to accept sickness as inevitable, the likelihood of their taking preventive action will be minimal. These responses, in turn, may be affected by any of the Cues to Action listed in the model. The conclusion, or outcome, of this blending of influences is a decision to either take the preventive action or not. As the model indicates, the decision that is reached will represent a weighing of the perceived benefits against the perceived barriers. The task of the change agent/planner will be to convince the target population that the benefits outweigh the barriers.

Lawrence Green, a prominent health educator, says that in order to bring about change, the change agent/planner needs to consider three groups of factors: *predisposing, enabling,* and *reinforcing. Predisposing* factors are those that motivate the target population to enter into the change transaction. To the target population they represent the *benefits* to be gained from making the proposed change. It is the task of the change agent/planner to convince them that the change will, in fact, bring about the benefits they have perceived. Once the target population has committed to making the change, the *enabling* factors come into play. These represent the *means* by which the perceived benefits will be realized. The efficient change agent/planner will have ensured beforehand that these means are available. That is, he or she will have made an accurate assessment of both the target population's abilities, need levels, and perceptions, as well as the availability of facilities and services, *before* embarking on the change transaction. *Reinforcing* factors are designed to insure maintenance of the new behavior, and come into play once the change has been made. Since it is hoped that the change will be long-term rather than a one-shot affair, it is important for the planner to build into his or her plan such *rewards* or *inducements* so the target population will maintain the new behavior. These may be either intrinsic or extrinsic in nature; in either case, they are designed to encourage the continuation of the new behavior.

Bandura's Self-Efficacy theory states that three types of expectancies underlie and determine behavior: (1) situation outcome, (2) action outcome, and (3) perceived self-efficacy. *Situation outcome* refers to assumptions about which consequences will occur, whether or not the recommended action is taken. For example, what is the likelihood of my developing cancer if I continue to smoke? Or, just how susceptible am I to the health threat? *Action outcome* refers to the belief that a given action will, or will not, lead to a specific consequence. For example, practicing abstinence will prevent my getting pregnant. *Self-efficacy* means that the recommended action either is or isn't within my ability to implement. The change agent needs to be aware of these expectancies, and prepared to deal with them in his or her program implementation plan.

It is important to note that because change of any kind requires effort on the part of the target population, it is often viewed as painful, unpleasant, and something to be resisted. This attitude may prevail even when the change is not only essential to the health and safety of the individual target, but of the entire community. In such a case, more stringent methods of gaining compliance may have to be resorted to. Herbert Kelman, a sociologist, suggests that at this point rules, regulations, and penalties for failing to follow them, need to be put in place. For parents, this means setting rules of conduct and behavior for the child, as well as a clear statement of consequences should they be broken. The rules should, of course, be tailored to the child's abilities, and the consequences in keeping with the seriousness of the noncompliant behavior and commensurate with the ability to enforce them. The same may be said for the schools and other community-based public sector resources. They have both the means and responsibility to establish and enforce standards of acceptable health behavior.

Government also plays a role in behavior change. Recent bans on smoking in selected public places, the seat belt law, speed limits on driving, and mandatory immunizations for school-age children prior to school entrance, are examples of governmental actions designed to protect the health and safety of the public. Kelman points out that this punitive approach is often a necessary first step to "unfreeze" behavior and bring about an immediate behavior change. The new behavior is likely to continue as long as the threat of punishment or blame remains; if it is maintained over time, it will become habitual. Once this occurs, the new behavior will have become an integral part of the target population's life-style—the ultimate goal of any behavior-change strategy.

SUMMARY

We have been looking at behavior change from the perspectives of the target population and the change agent/planner. The target population may be a single individual, a group, or an entire community. The change agent/planner may be a parent, teacher, health professional, organization, or government. Regardless of who they are, education and compliance should be the primary focuses of their health behavior change strategy to prevent disease. Education brings the disease-prevention message to the target population—an essential first step. However, education alone will not necessarily lead to the target population's taking appropriate action with respect to disease prevention. To motivate this action, a variety of behavior-change strategies need to be applied. It is the change agent/planner's responsibility to select those strategies that best fit the characteristics and needs of the target population, based on a needs assessment and the factors underlying behavior.

LEARNING OBJECTIVES

From the information included in this chapter, the student will be able to:

1. explain why information giving/education is a necessary first step in changing behavior.
2. explain why information giving/education alone is usually ineffective in changing behavior.
3. tell why the home and school are good starting points for inculcating positive health behaviors.
4. explain what a school health council is, and list three functions of the council.
5. distinguish between the public and private sectors, and give an example of an organization for each sector.
6. define the terms: *ownership; change agent;* and *voluntary health agency.*
7. explain Maslow's Hierarchy of Needs theory.
8. tell how Maslow's theory might be used by the change agent.
9. explain Edward Hall's theory.
10. tell how Hall's theory might be used by the change agent.
11. tell what a needs assessment is and what its purposes are.

REFERENCES

Bloom, M. *Primary Prevention Practices.* Thousand Oaks, CA: Sage Publications, 1996.

Butler, J. T. *Principles of Health Education and Health Promotion.* Englewood, CO: Morton Publishing Co., 1994.

Conner, M., and P. Norman, eds. *Predicting Health Behavior.* Buckingham, U.K.: Open University Press, 1996.

Gochman, D. S., ed. *Health Behavior.* New York: Plenum Press, 1988.

Green, L., and M. W. Kreuter. *Health Promotion Planning.* Mountain View, CA: Mayfield Publishing Co., 1991.

Hall, E. T. *The Silent Language.* New York: Doubleday and Co., 1959.

Kelman, H. "Compliance, Identification and Internalization." P. 444 in *The Planning of Change.* New York: Holt, Rinehart and Winston, 1961.

Koop, C. E. "Editorial: A Personal Role in Health Cure Reform." *AJPH* 85: 759, 1995.

Lewin, K., T. Dembo, L. Festinger, and P. S. Sears. "Level of Aspiration." Pp. 333–78 in *Personality and Behavior Disorders.* New York: Ronald Press, 1944.

McKenzie, J. F., and J. Jurs. *Planning, Implementing, and Evaluating Health Promotion Programs*. New York: Macmillan Publishing Co., 1993.

Rosenstock, I. M., V. J. Strecher, and M. H. Becker. "Social Learning Theory and The Health Belief Model." *Health Education Quarterly* 15: 175–83, 1988.

Timmreck, T. C. *Program Planning, Development and Evaluation*. Boston: Jones and Bartlett, 1995.

Witkin, B. R., and J. W. Altschuld. *Planning and Conducting Needs Assessments*. Thousand Oaks, CA: Sage Publications, 1995.

APPENDIX: PROBLEMS

PROBLEM 1

Beginning in the mid-70s and continuing to today, the incidence of tuberculosis in New York City has escalated to almost epidemic proportions. This occurrence has been attributed to a variety of factors, all of which have compounded the problem. Some of these are: AIDS, an influx of immigrants, housing overcrowding, massive elimination of low-income housing, a rise in illicit drug use, and homelessness. Many of the immigrants coming to New York City had been vaccinated against tuberculosis prior to their arrival. It was later learned, however, that the vaccine they received had passed its expiration date and was, therefore, ineffective. In addition to not protecting against the disease, the vaccine produced a false reading on tuberculin exposure tests, making it difficult to ascertain whether a person was, in fact, harboring a case of tuberculosis.

1. Identify the health problem in the above paragraph.
2. To which category of communicable diseases does tuberculosis belong?
3. Classify the factors mentioned in the paragraph as to whether they are social, biological, or environmental.
4. Explain how each may have contributed to the problem.
5. Using the information given in the paragraph, trace the natural history of tuberculosis from prepathogenesis through pathogenesis. Cite from the paragraph specific examples to support your answer.

PROBLEM 2

In a study reported in the *American Journal of Public Health*[1] it was stated that African Americans have a longer delay time in seeking care for acute heart problems, in spite of the fact that this population also has higher morbidity and mortality rates from heart disease than U.S. whites.

Reasons given for the delay in seeking care include: (1) lack of health insurance; (2) lack of a regular source of health care; (3) dissatisfaction with previous encounters with health care-givers; (4) lack of information; (5) lack of transportation; (6) depending on a family member to seek help; (7) intermittent, nonincapacitating pain, rather than persistent, severe pain; (8) living alone; and (9) attempts at self-treatment. Severity of pain and having a history of heart problems were identified as reasons for seeking help more promptly.

1. Categorize each of the reasons reported, both for delaying and not delaying, according to the divisions of the Health Belief Model, i.e., Individual Perceptions, Modifying Factors, and Likelihood of Action.
2. For each of the first five reasons listed in the paragraph, mention a way of removing it as a barrier to seeking care.
3. Indicate whether this removal is the responsibility of the individual, the community, or the government, and justify your answers.

---

1. Ell, Kathleen, et al. "Acute Chest Pain in African Americans: Factors in the Delay in Seeking Emergency Care." *AJPH* 84: 965–70, 1994.

PROBLEM 3

Approximately 13 million Americans have been diagnosed as having diabetes mellitus, the seventh leading cause of death in the United States. Of these, Hispanics, African Americans, and Native Americans have significantly higher prevalence rates for this disease. This phenomenon has been associated with late detection; since the complications resulting from diabetes mellitus are serious, early diagnosis is of prime importance.

1. What is meant by the term, *prevalence rate?*
2. From your knowledge of diabetes mellitus, what reasons can you infer for the high prevalence rate among the ethnic groups mentioned in the paragraph?
3. Suggest one predisposing factor that might be employed to encourage early detection.
4. Suggest one enabling factor that might be employed with respect to detection.
5. Suggest one reinforcing factor that might be employed with respect to detection.
6. For each answer to questions 3, 4, and 5, indicate whether the individual, community, or government is responsible for implementation.

PROBLEM 4

The prevalence of hepatitis B infection (HBV) has become a major health problem in the United States. The following groups have been identified as high-risk with respect to HBV infection: health care workers; hemophiliacs; hemodialysis patients; sex partners of HBV-positive people; injection drug users; sexually active individuals who have more than one sex partner; inmates of long-term correctional institutions.[2]

1. With respect to hepatitis B, what is the common link shared by the high-risk groups mentioned in the paragraph?
2. For each group, identify a primary prevention activity that could break the chain of infection.
3. For each group, identify a secondary prevention activity that could break the chain of infection.
4. For one primary prevention activity, identify predisposing, enabling, and reinforcing factors that could encourage implementation of the activity.
5. Identify the same factors for one secondary prevention activity.

---

2. Adapted from Advisory Committee on Immunization Practices (ACIP). "Hepatitis B Virus: A Comprehensive Strategy for Eliminating Transmission in the United States Through Universal Childhood Vaccination." *MMWR* 40 (RR–13): 1–25, 1991.

PROBLEM 5

In spite of the fact that she had been diagnosed with systemic lupus erythematosus, a young woman had succeeded in earning a place on her college's varsity swim team. For several years, her condition had been kept in remission by ongoing medical intervention and monitoring. In her senior year, however, she began to show signs of chronic renal failure, which necessitated her being placed in dialysis. Despite the dialysis, her condition deteriorated to the point where she was on the verge of a coma. Nevertheless, she persisted in her belief that she would recover, be able to return to college and even the swim team. She described herself as the sort of person who could do anything once she made up her mind to do it. She was confident that she would recover quickly from this episode once the correct combination of drugs was found.

1. Name the health problem and which disease group it belongs to.
2. Justify your classification, and include the name of the body system most intimately involved in this disease.
3. Apply the Health Belief Model by citing examples from the paragraph of: (a) the patient's perceptions of her condition and prognosis, and (b) modifying factors and cues to action.

PROBLEM 6

A teenage single, expectant mother in her last month of pregnancy collapses on the street and is rushed to the nearest emergency room. There she is diagnosed as suffering from severe preeclampsia, a condition related to pregnancy and characterized by hypertension, fluid retention, spillage of protein into the urine, dizziness, and headaches. When she regains consciousness, the emergency room physician tells her she must stay in the hospital throughout the rest of her pregnancy for her own health and that of the child she is carrying. She responds to the physician's advice by declaring that she got through to this stage of the pregnancy without anyone's help, and she doesn't want any now.

1. What primary preventive measure has been lacking throughout this pregnancy?
2. What secondary preventive measure is being suggested in the paragraph?
3. List three possible reasons for this teenager's failure to practice primary prevention during her pregnancy.
4. List three ways in which either the community and/or government might have enabled this teenager to practice primary prevention.

PROBLEM 7

In the aftermath of the 1991 measles epidemic in New York City, a study was made of vaccination rates of children enrolled in WIC programs and children whose health care providers were private physicians.[3] The study revealed that WIC-enrolled children were at a 32 percent higher risk of contracting measles for lack of vaccination, while children under the care of a private physician were at a 20 percent risk.

1. From the paragraph, what reasons can you infer for: (a) the discrepancy in risk levels between the two groups of children, and (b) the fact that 20 percent of the children with private physicians were unvaccinated?
2. How does vaccination intervene in the disease process?
3. To which of the body's lines of defense does vaccination apply?
4. Which kind of immunity does vaccination confer?
5. Identify one benefit and one drawback of this kind of immunity.

---

3. LeBaron, Charles W., et al. "Measles Vaccination Levels of Children Enrolled in WIC during the 1991 Measles Epidemic in New York City." *AJPH* 86: 1551–56, 1996.

PROBLEM 8

Data collected in the 1985 National Nursing Home Survey were analyzed to identify risk factors for infections and mortality.[4] Pneumonia and urinary tract infections were the conditions found to be most prevalent among the nursing home residents studied. Rates of infection for both these conditions were significantly higher among bed-bound patients, those who were incontinent for both bowel and urine, and those requiring indwelling catheterization.

1. From the paragraph, identify the risk factors mentioned for pneumonia and urinary tract infections, and explain why they are contributing factors to these conditions.
2. Which categories of communicable disease do pneumonia and urinary tract infections belong to? Explain your choice of classification.
3. Show how each of the three Biological Laws of Disease may be applied to the Nursing Home Survey data.

4. Hing, E., et al. "National Nursing Home Survey: 1985 Summary for United States." *Vital Health Statistics* 13: 97, 1989. DHHS publication PHS 89: 1758.

PROBLEM 9

One of the fastest growing health problems in the Middle Atlantic states is Lyme disease, a vector-borne disease. A burgeoning deer population in the area has been identified as the primary reason for this increase in incidence. Deer prefer to live in thickly wooded areas which offer them an ample food supply; such areas are also regarded as desirable habitats by people. As a result, deer and humans live in close proximity to each other, thus increasing the possibility that the human will come into contact with the vector. In the case of Lyme disease, the vector is a tick carried on the body of the deer, which may pass onto shrubbery as the deer forages for food. Then, when a person passes through the same area, the tick may attach itself to the person and bite him or her, thereby transfering the spirochete which causes Lyme disease.

1. Which of the body's lines of defense is breached in the transmission of Lyme disease?
2. To which category of communicable disease does Lyme disease belong?
3. What is meant by incidence of Lyme disease?
4. From the paragraph, what inferences can you draw as to what the roles of the individual and the community might be in reducing the incidence of this disease?
5. Apply the Health Belief Model to this problem from the perspectives of both the individual and community.

PROBLEM 10

Childhood asthma and lead poisoning continue to be two major health concerns, in spite of the fact that much is known about the factors contributing to their occurrence, and also that we have the ability to either eliminate or control many of them. Some of the factors contributing to childhood asthma include: exposure to side-stream smoke from parents or care-takers, exposure to stress, exposure to environmental pollutants, crowded living conditions, homelessness, and poor nutrition. Childhood lead poisoning has been attributed to the presence of lead-based paint on the walls of dwellings, as well as on toys and other objects that a child may try to put in his or her mouth. It has also been attributed to prolonged exposure to airborne lead that may result from vehicle emissions and/or construction work.

1. Identify which group of diseases childhood asthma and lead poisoning belong to.
2. Show how the three Biological Laws of Disease may be applied to both diseases.
3. For each disease, list steps that the individual might take to either prevent or minimize the likelihood of its developing.
4. For each disease, list steps that might be taken by the community and/or government to prevent or minimize the likelihood of its developing.

GLOSSARY

acquired characteristics. Characteristics for which there is no genetic marker, and which develop after the delivery of the baby.

active immunity. The type of immunity that results when the body produces its own antibodies in response to an antigen.

adrenaline. A hormone released by the adrenal glands when the body is faced with a threat, either real or imagined. Also known as **epinephrine**.

agent. The cause of a communicable disease; is always a **germ** or **pathogen**.

agglutination. One of the antibody responses to an antigen.

air sacs. Located in the lungs, and act as the exchange stations for oxygen and carbon dioxide between the lungs and the blood. Also known as **alveoli**.

Alzheimer's disease. A non-communicable disease associated with aging.

amino acids. The basic ingredient of protein.

amniocentesis. A test given to pregnant women to identify possible fetal problems.

amyotropic lateral sclerosis. Also known as Lou Gehrig's disease, a non-communicable disease characterized by progressive inability of the muscles to function.

antibodies. Protein elements which react only against the antigen responsible for their production.

antigen. Any foreign element that stimulates the body to produce its own antibodies.

antigenicity. A pathogen characteristic; the ability to stimulate the body to produce antibodies.

arteries. One type of blood vessel; always carry blood away from the heart.

arterioles. The smallest arteries in the body.

arteriosclerosis. A condition in which the arteries become less elastic; a normal concomitant of aging.

arthritis. Inflammation of the joints of the body.

arthropods. Parasites living on the surface of the host's body.

asthma. A non-communicable disease characterized by episodes of breathing difficulty.

atherosclerosis. A non-communicable disease related to the accumulation of plaque on the inner walls of the arteries.

atria. The upper, or receiving, chambers of the heart. Also known as **auricles**.

atrioventricular node. One of the nerve bundles in the heart that regulate the rate of its contractions.

bacillus. The rod-shaped form of bacteria.

bacteria. One group of pathogens that promote disease in man.

benign tumor. A noncancerous growth of cells.

bicuspid valve. A structure in the left side of the heart that permits blood to flow from the left atrium into the left ventricle.

Biological Laws of Disease. Three canons that explain the way in which disease develops.

blood. The transport medium of the body.

blood pressure. A measure of the force with which the heart must contract in order to circulate blood around the body.

bronchi. Two passages in the lungs through which air passes, both into and out of the body. Also known as **bronchial tubes**.

bronchioles. The smallest branches of the bronchi.

Bundle of His. A nerve bundle in the heart that regulates the rate of contraction of the heart.

cancer. A non-communicable disease characterized by a proliferation of cells which perform no useful function, usurp the space and food supply of normal cells, and have the ability to spread to other sites in the body.

capillaries. The smallest blood vessels in the body; serve as exchange stations between the cells and the blood.

carbohydrates. One of the essential nutrients; made of carbon, hydrogen, and oxygen.

carcinogen. A cancer-inducing substance.

carcinoma. One of the major types of cancer.

cerebral palsy. A non-communicable disease involving the central nervous system.

cerebrovascular disease. Also known as **stroke**; a non-communicable disease in which a clot lodges in the brain.

cholesterol. A fatty substance produced by the body and intimately involved in the development of plaque in atherosclerosis.

chorionic villus analysis. A test given to pregnant women to identify possible fetal problems.

chromosomes. The carriers of the genes; humans have twenty-three pairs.

chronic bronchitis. A non-communicable disease involving inflammation of the bronchi.

chronic occupational pulmonary disease. Also known as **COPD**; a group of non-communicable diseases resulting from prolonged exposure to respiratory tract irritants.

cilia. Tiny hairs lining the respiratory passages and designed to filter out foreign matter from the air that we inhale.

clinical horizon. An imaginary line separating the early stages of pathogenesis from later stages in which signs and symptoms become apparent.

coccus. A ball or spherical-shaped form of bacteria.

communicable disease. Also known as **infectious disease**; always involves a susceptible host, a causative agent, or germ, and a mode of transmission.

congenital. Refers to a condition that arises in the fetus during the gestation period; has no genetic marker.

connective tissue. The tissue that attaches one part of the body to another; also refers to ligaments and tendons surrounding the joints of the body.

contact. One of the communicable disease groupings. Also known as **integumentary.**

coronary heart disease. Also known as **ischemic heart disease**; a leading cause of death in the United States.

dermotropic. A type of virus.

diabetes mellitus. A non-communicable disease resulting from insufficient production of insulin by the islet cells of the pancreas.

diabetic coma. A condition that arises when there is insufficient insulin to enable the body to metabolize carbohydrates.

diastolic pressure. One of the measurable blood pressures; an index of arterial resistance to the flow of blood.

diffusion. A process whereby substances pass through a semipermeable membrane from an area of greater concentration to an area of lesser concentration.

Down's syndrome. A condition arising from a chromosomal defect.

embolus. A moving clot.

endemic. A term used to describe a disease or condition that is common to a specific geographic area.

endocrine glands. Glands which secrete their hormones directly into the bloodstream.

epidemic. A term used to describe an outbreak of a disease, in which the number of new cases exceeds the number that is expected.

epilepsy. An intermittent brain disorder occurring mostly in males.

epinephrine. Another name for **adrenalin**, one of the adrenal gland hormones.

essential hypertension. High blood pressure for which there is no known cause.

fats. One of the nutrients needed by the body.

fomite. An inanimate object that carries disease agents.

fungi. A group of organisms that is capable of producing disease in man.

genetic. A term used to describe a characteristic that is determined by a gene.

genetic makeup. A term that describes the full complement of a person's inherited traits.

germ. A disease-causing agent; a pathogen.

glucose. A simple sugar; the principal source of energy for the body.

gout. A non-communicable joint disease that principally affects the big toe.

Health Belief Model. A paradigm for understanding health behavior.

heart attack. A life-threatening occurrence in which the heart malfunctions.

heart murmur. A condition in which the valves of the heart fail to close completely, allowing seepage of blood between atrium and ventricle.

heart rate. Also known as **pulse rate**; the rate at which the heart contracts.

helminths. disease-producing worms.

hemoglobin. The oxygen-carrying component of the blood.

hemophilia. An inherited disorder in which the blood lacks the elements needed for clotting.

histiocytes. Phagocytic cells of the bone marrow and spleen.

homeostasis. A state of the body in which all systems are in equilibrium.

hormones. Chemical substances secreted by endocrine glands to regulate body processes.

host. The recipient or target of the disease causing agent or risk factor.

hyperglycemia. A condition in which the glucose concentration of the blood has risen above what is considered normal.

hyperthyroidism. A condition in which too much thyroxin is produced.

hypoglycemia. A condition in which too little glucose is present in the blood.

hypotension. Low blood pressure.

hypothyroidism. A condition in which an insufficient quantity of thyroxin is present in the blood.

incidence. The number of new cases of a disease occurring since a designated date.

incubation period. The time during the pathogenesis period when the disease-producing agent is lodging, multiplying, and spreading.

infectivity. A pathogen characteristic related to its ability to lodge, multiply, and spread.

ingestion. The process whereby we take in food and drink.

inhalation. The process whereby we take in air.

inherited characteristics. Characteristics determined by genes at the moment of conception.

insulin. The hormone released by the islet cells of the pancreas, which is essential for the metabolism of carbohydrates.

insulin-dependent diabetes mellitus. Also known as Type I diabetes; requires lifelong administration of insulin.

insulin shock. A life-threatening condition in which too much insulin is in the blood at a given time.

interferon. A component of the reticulo-endothelial system, and part of the body's second line of defense.

iodine. A mineral needed in the formation of thyroxin by the thyroid gland.

iron. A mineral needed by the body for the formation of hemoglobin, the oxygen-carrying component of the blood.

iron deficiency anemia. A condition in which the body is unable to produce hemoglobin because of an iron-poor diet.

joint. The meeting, or articulation, of two bones.

lead poisoning. A condition in which the concentration of lead in the blood exceeds acceptable levels.

leukemia. A form of cancer in which the white blood cells proliferate.

leukocytes. Another name for white blood cells.

Lyme disease. A vector-borne, integumentary disease.

lymphatic system. An auxiliary circulatory system designed to drain off wastes from the cells.

lymphomas. One of the major types of cancer.

lysis. One of the ways antibodies respond to antigens.

macrophages. Phagocytic cells that are part of the reticulo-endothelial system.

malignant tumors. Another term for cancerous growths.

melanomas. One of the major types of cancer.

metastasis. The ability of a cancer cell to break away from the original growth to form a new colony in another part of the body.

monocytes. Another term for leukocytes.

morbidity rate. A ratio comparing the number of people in a given community who are ill with a specific disease at a specific time, with the total number of people living in the community at the same time.

mortality rate. A ratio comparing the number of people in a given community who die at a specific time, with the total number of people living there at the same time.

mucous membranes. Tissues lining all body cavities.

mucus. The sticky substance released by mucous membranes which lubricates the lining and prevents foreign matter from penetrating the body further.

multiple sclerosis. A central nervous system disorder.

muscular dystrophy. A group of diseases characterized by progressive muscle wasting and weakness.

mycoses. The group of diseases caused by fungi.

myocardial infarction. A heart attack.

natural history of disease. The progression of a disease from pre-pathogenesis through pathogenesis.

neutralization. One of the ways in which antibodies respond to antigens.

noninsulin-dependent diabetes mellitus. Also known as Type II diabetes; can be managed by means of diet, exercise, and weight control.

opsonization. One of the ways in which antibodies respond to antigens.

osteoarthritis. A disease in which the joints have become eroded.

pacemaker. Also known as the sinoatrial node; regulates the rate of the heartbeat.

pandemic. A term used to describe a disease that occurs everywhere in the world.

parasitic. The state in which an organism derives all of its food from another.

Parkinson's disease. A central nervous system disorder.

pathogen. A germ; the causative agent of a communicable disease.

pathogenesis. A period in the natural history of a disease.

pathogenicity. A pathogen characteristic; the ability of the pathogen to create a disease state in the host.

period of communicability. The time during which a disease may be spread from one source to another.

pernicious anemia. A non-communicable disease in which insufficient red blood cells are produced.

phagocytosis. The process whereby white cells, lymph cells and antibodies destroy foreign substances that have entered the body.

phenylketonuria. A disorder in which the body is incapable of metabolizing protein.

phlebitis. A condition in which a clot lodges in a blood vessel in the leg.

phosphorus. A mineral needed by the body for growth of bones and teeth.

plaque. Term used to describe the accumulation of cholesterol deposits on the inner walls of the arteries.

plasma. The liquid portion of the blood.

platelets. The clotting elements of the blood.

pneumotropic. Term used to describe a group of viruses.

precipitating factor. Also known as a risk factor, makes the host more prone to a disease.

precipitation. One way in which antibodies respond to an antigen.

prematurity. When a baby weighs less than 2,500 grams, or 5½ pounds at birth.

prepathogenesis. The stage in the natural history of a disease in which the host and agent come together.

prevalence. The total number of cases of a disease at a given time.

primary prevention. The steps taken before the fact to keep from contracting an illness.

proteins. One of the nutrients needed by the body for growth and repair.

protozoa. A group of disease-producing organisms in man.

pulmonary artery. The artery that carries deoxygenated blood from the heart to the lungs.

pulmonary vein. The vein that carries oxygenated blood from the lungs to the heart.

red blood cells. Also known as **erythrocytes**; their function is to carry food and oxygen to the cells.

reflexes. Automatic responses to stimuli.

reservoir. A breeding place for pathogens.

reticulo-endothelial system. One of the body's second-line defenses; made up of histiocytes, leukocytes, macrophages, and interferon.

rheumatoid arthritis. A joint disorder marked by swelling, tenderness, and pain.

rickettsia. A group of disease-producing organisms in man.

sarcomas. A major type of cancer.

secondary prevention. Also known as after-the-fact care; steps taken in response to an illness.

septum. The wall separating the right side of the heart from the left.

serum. A substance containing antibodies made outside of the host's body and injected into him or her for the purpose of conferring passive immunity.

sickle-cell disease. A genetically transmitted blood disease in which the red cells assume a sickle shape.

sign. An objective measure or indicator of disease.

sinoatrial node. A bundle of nerve fibers that regulate the rate of contraction of the heart.

skin. The outermost line of defense against pathogens.

sodium. A mineral needed by the body for the maintenance of normal homeostasis.

spirochete. A type of bacteria characterized by its corkscrew shape.

staphylococcus. A ball or spherical-shaped bacteria.

stimulant. Any substance that increases blood pressure, heart and breathing rates, and temperature; preparing the body to take action against a threat.

streptococcus. A form of bacteria.

stroke. A condition arising when a clot lodges in a blood vessel in the brain and impedes blood circulation to that part of the brain; the part of the body controlled by the affected section of the brain becomes paralyzed.

susceptible host. A person whose resistance level is too low to enable him or her to ward off an attacking pathogen.

symptom. A subjective indication of illness, one that cannot be measured quantitatively.

synovial fluid. Fluid found within the synovial membrane of a joint; its purpose is to lubricate the joint.

synovial membrane. The membrane which contains the synovial fluid.

systemic lupus erythematosus. An inflammatory, autoimmune disease affecting many parts of the body.

systolic pressure. The pressure exerted by the heart as it contracts; the numerator in a blood pressure reading.

tertiary prevention. Another term for rehabilitation.

thrombus. A lodged clot.

trachea. The windpipe.

tricuspid valve. Situated on the right side of the heart; controls the flow of blood from the right atrium into the right ventricle.

trophozoite. The active stage in the life cycle of a protozoa.

tropism. A characteristic of viruses, enabling them to attach themselves to receptors.

ultrasound scanning. A test given to a pregnant woman to identify possible fetal problems.

vaccination. The act of administering a vaccine; used in conferring active immunity.

vector. An animate object which carries a pathogen; examples are fleas, ticks, and mosquitoes.

veins. Blood vessels which always carry blood to the heart.

vena cava. Superior and inferior vena cava—the two largest veins in the body—collect deoxygenated blood from the upper and lower parts of the body, respectively, and deposit it in the right atrium.

ventricles. The lower or discharging chambers of the heart.

virulence. A pathogen characteristic referring to its potency.

viruses. The smallest pathogens that attack man.

viscerotropic. A class of viruses.

BIBLIOGRAPHY

Advisory Committee on Immunization Practices (ACIP). "Hepatitis B Virus: A Comprehensive Strategy for Eliminating Transmission in the United States Through Universal Childhood Vaccination." *MMWR* 40 (RR–13): 1–25, 1991.

Becker, M., ed. *The Health Belief Model and Personal Health Behavior.* Thoroughfare, NJ: Slack, 1974.

Benenson, A. S., ed. *Control of Communicable Disease Manual.* 16th ed. Washington, DC: American Public Health Association, 1996.

Bickley, H. C. *Practical Concepts in Human Disease.* 2d ed. Baltimore: Williams and Wilkins, 1977.

Bloom, M. *Primary Prevention Practices.* Thousand Oaks, CA: Sage Publications, 1996.

Brooks, S. M. *Basic Facts of Medical Microbiology.* Philadelphia: W. B. Saunders Company, 1962.

Brownson, R. C., P. L. Remington, and J. R. Davis, eds. *Chronic Disease Epidemiology and Control.* Washington, DC: American Public Health Association, 1993.

Butler, J. T. *Principles of Health Education and Health Promotion.* Englewood, CO: Morton Publishing Co., 1994.

Campbell, J. "Making Sense of Immunity and Immunization." *Nursing Times* 90: 32–34, 1994.

Ciesielski, P. F. *Major Chronic Diseases.* Guilford, CT: The Dushkin Publishing Group, 1992.

Conner, M., and P. Norman, eds. *Predicting Health Behavior.* Buckingham, U.K.: Open University Press, 1996.

Crowley, L. V. *Introduction to Human Disease.* 4th ed. Boston: Jones and Bartlett, 1996.

Dickey, L. L., H. M. Griffith, and D. B. Kamerow. "Put Prevention Into Practice." In *Clinician's Handbook of Preventive Services*. U.S. Department of Health and Human Services. PHS, Office of Disease Prevention and Health Promotion, 1994.

Edelson, P. J. "Editorial: The Need for Innovation in Immunization." *AJPH* 85: 1613, 1995.

Edlin, G., E. Golanty, and K. McCormack Brown. *Health and Wellness*. 5th ed. Boston: Jones and Bartlett Publishers, 1996.

Ell, K., et al. "Acute Chest Pain in African Americans: Factors in the Delay in Seeking Emergency Care." *AJPH* 84: 965–70, 1994.

Evans, A. S., and P. S. Brachman. *Bacterial Infections of Humans: Epidemiology and Control*. 2d. ed. New York: Plenum Medical Book Co., 1991.

Fairbrother, G., and K. A. DuMont. "New York City's Child Immunization Day: Planning, Costs, and Results." *AJPH* 85: 1662–65, 1995.

Fardy, P. S., J. Magel, and M. Hurster, et al. "Prevalence of Coronary Artery Disease Risk Factors in Minority Adolescents: A Feasibility Study." *J. Cardiopulmonary Rehab*. 9: 404, 1989.

Fardy, P. S., R. E. C. White, L. T. Clark, and M. Hurster, et al. "Coronary Risk Factors and Health Behaviors in a Diverse Ethnic and Cultural Population of Adolescents: A Gender Comparison." *J. Cardiopulmonary Rehab*. 14: 52–60, 1994.

———. "Health Promotion in Minority Adolescents." *J. Cardiopulmonary Rehab*. 15: 65–72, 1995.

Gochman, D. S., ed. *Health Behavior*. New York: Plenum Press, 1988.

Green, L., and M. W. Kreuter. *Health Promotion Planning*. 2nd ed. Mountain View, CA: Mayfield Publishing Company, 1991.

Guyton, A. C., and J. E. Hall. *Textbook of Medical Physiology*. 9th ed. Philadelphia: W. B. Saunders Company, 1995.

Hall, E. T. *The Silent Language*. New York: Doubleday and Co., 1959.

Hing, E., et al. "National Nursing Home Survey: 1985 Summary for the United States." *Vital Health Statistics* 13: 97, 1989. DHHS Publication PHS 89: 1758.

Kandel, D., P. Wu, and M. Davies. "Maternal Smoking During Pregnancy and Smoking by Adolescent Daughters." *AJPH* 84: 1407–13, 1994.

Kelman, H. "Compliance, Identification and Internalization." P. 444 in *The Planning of Change*. New York: Holt, Rinehart and Winston, 1961.

Kerson, T. S., and L. A. Kerson. *Understanding Chronic Illness*. New York: The Free Press, 1985.

Koop, C. E. "Editorial: A Personal Role in Health Care Reform." *AJPH* 85: 759, 1995.

Kotelchuck, M. "The Adequacy of Prenatal Care Utilization Index: Its U.S.

Distribution and Association with Low Birthweight." *AJPH* 84: 1486–88, 1994.

Krebs-Smith, S. M., A. Cook, and A. Subar, et al. "U.S. Adults' Fruit and Vegetable Intakes, 1989 to 1991: A Revised Baseline for the Healthy People 2000 Objective." *AJPH* 85: 1623–28, 1995.

Krieger, N. "Analyzing Socioeconomic Patterns in Health and Health Care." *AJPH* 83: 1086–87, 1993.

Land, G. H., and J. W. Stockbauer. "Smoking and Pregnancy Outcome: Trends Among Black Teenage Mothers in Missouri." *AJPH* 83: 1121–24, 1993.

LeBaron, C. W., et al. "Measles Vaccination Levels of Children Enrolled in WIC During the 1991 Measles Epidemic in New York City." *AJPH* 86: 1551–56, 1996.

Lewin, K., T. Dembo, L. Festinger, and P. S. Sears. "Level of Aspiration." Pp. 333–78 in *Personality and Behavior Disorders*. New York: Ronald Press, 1944.

Lewy, R. *Preventive Primary Medicine*. Boston: Little, Brown, 1980.

Mandell, G. L., R. G. Douglas, Jr., and J. E. Bennett, eds. *Principles and Practices of Infectious Diseases*. 3d ed. New York: Churchill Livingstone, 1992.

Marshall, J. "Editorial: Improving Americans' Diet—Setting Public Policy with Limited Knowledge." *AJPH* 85: 1609–10, 1995.

McKenzie, J. F., and J. Jurs. *Planning, Implementing, and Evaluating Health Promotion Programs*. New York: Macmillan Publishing Co., 1993.

Public Health Service. "Healthy People 2000. National Health Promotion and Prevention Objectives." Washington, DC: U.S. Department of Health and Human Services, 1991. DHHS Publication PHS 91: 50212.

Purtilo, D. T., and R. B. Purtilo. *A Survey of Human Diseases*. Boston: Little, Brown Co., 1989.

Rosenstock, I. M., V. J. Strecher, and M. H. Becker. "Social Learning Theory and The Health Belief Model." *Health Education Quarterly* 15: 175–83, 1988.

Shea, S. "Editorial: Hypertension Control." *AJPH* 84: 1725–26, 1994.

Sheldon, H. *Boyd's Introduction to the Study of Disease*. Philadelphia: Lea & Febiger, 1984.

Smith, D. T., N. F. Conant, and J. R. Overman. *Zinnser Microbiology*. 13th ed. New York: Appleton-Century-Crofts, 1964.

Timmreck, T. C. *An Introduction to Epidemiology*. Boston: Jones & Bartlett, 1994.

———. *Program Planning, Development and Evaluation*. Boston: Jones & Bartlett, 1995.

Waisbren, S. E., and B. D. Hamilton, et al. "Psychosocial Factors in Maternal Phenylketonuria: Women's Adherence to Medical Recommendations." *AJPH* 85: 1636–40, 1995.

Witkin, B. R., and J. W. Altschuld. *Planning and Conducting Needs Assessments.* Thousand Oaks, CA: Sage Publications, 1995.

INDEX

Cilia, 1, 7
Cleft palate, 46, 96
Clinical horizon, 17
Clots, 60–61
Common cold, 31
Communicability, period of, 19
Communicable disease: categories
    of, 31; defined, 25
Compliance, 109
Congenital characteristics, 46
Congenital herpes simplex, 46
Conjunctivitis, 31
Contact diseases, 29, 31
Coronary artery disease, 60
Coronary heart disease, 60
Cortisone, 74

Diabetes, 46; insipidus, 74; melli-
    tus, 75, 77, 78
Diabetic coma, 87
Diastolic blood pressure, 53
Diffusion, 51
Disease agent, 3
Down's syndrome, 46, 95

Embolus, 61
Emphysema, 63
Endemic, 18
Endocrine glands, 73
Environmental hazards, 44
Epidemic, 18
Epilepsy, 83
Epinephrine, 57, 74

Festinger's Cognitive Dissonance
    theory, 114
Fetal alcohol syndrome, 46, 96
Fight or flight response, 111
Fomite, 33
Food, functions of, 86
Food Guide Pyramid, 85
Fungi, 28

Genetic makeup, 43
Genetic risk factor, 4
Glomerulonephritis, 10
Gonads, 73, 75
Gonorrhea, 36, 46
Gout, 81
Green's behavioral factors theory,
    117, 118

Hall's stages of conditioning theory,
    113–114
Health Belief Model, 115, 117
Heart: attack, 60; murmur, 49; rate,
    51; related diseases, 48; structure,
    49
Helminths, 28
Hemophilia, 46, 95
Hepatitis A, 31, 37
Hepatitis B, 31, 35
Homeostasis, 89
Hormones, defined, 73
Host, 19
Hyper and hypo as prefixes, 75
Hyperglycemia, 87
Hypoglycemia, 87
Hypothalamus, 73

Immunotherapy, 73
Incidence, 18
Incubation period, 17, 19
Infectivity, 5, 25
Influenza, 31
Ingestion, 31
Inhalation, 29
Inherited characteristics, 45–46
Instinct, 111
Insulin shock, 87
Integumentary diseases, 31
Interferon, 8
Iodine, 92
Iron, 92

About the Author

MADELINE M. HURSTER is Retired Associate Professor of Health at Queens College, New York. She has served as Coordinator of the college's Health Education Program and has held offices in several professional health organizations. She is the author of numerous articles as well as the text, *Health for Better Living* (1964).

CPSIA information can be obtained at www.ICGtesting.com
Printed in the USA
LVOW13*0528100414

381077LV00005B/25/P